AF884940

MedStrong WORKBOOK

SHED YOUR MEDS FOR A BETTER, HEALTHIER YOU

AGING WELL THROUGH DEPRESCRIBING

5-Step Medication Optimization Plan

DONNA BARTLETT, PharmD, BCGP

MedStrong Workbook:
Shed Your Meds for a Better, Healthier You

By Donna Bartlett, PharmD, BCGP

This workbook includes information from many resources; however, it does not replace information on your health decisions between you and your health-care providers. This workbook does not diagnose or decide if a medication is the right medication for you and is not a substitute for making decisions with your health-care team. Use this workbook to assist with communication with your health-care providers to make the best decision for your health. The workbook is sold with the understanding that neither the author nor the publisher is rendering or substituting legal, medical, psychological, or physiological advice. The author and publisher disclaim any personal liability, directly or indirectly, for advice or information presented within. Although the author and publisher have diligently written and produced this workbook for accuracy and completeness of the information contained within, we assume no responsibility for errors, inaccuracies, omissions, inconsistencies, or changes in treatment.

Design: Chris Molé, Book Savvy Studio

ISBN 978-1-7377563-2-3
HEALTH / Medicine

For more information please contact the publisher at
WELLhood Publishing,
11 Brooks Road, Paxton, Massachusetts 01612 508-450-0269
Email: info@wellhoodpublishing.com

*To all the women and men who find themselves as caregivers, navigating the maze of health care and medications. Let's change the narrative by bringing the process to your fingertips. Become **MedStrong!***

"Deprescribing is not an easy undertaking, but it is a necessary task that healthcare professionals need to be proficient at in order to promote person-centered care. Dr. Bartlett's book is an amazing resource that provides a logical roadmap on how to approach optimizing a patient's medication regimen. The book offers many practical tools to enhance communication and patient education that foster a shared decision-making approach to deprescribing medications that no longer provide clinical advantages and may likely detract from quality of life. Our goal as healthcare professionals should be to provide our patients with the best care possible, and there comes a point in a patient's healthcare journey where doing less is more."

~ ANDY ARWARI, MD, MS, FACP, SFHM, FAAHPM, HMDC

Acknowledgements

THERE ARE SO MANY that have continued on the *MedStrong* journey with me! They have embraced the importance of *MedStrong*—that is deprescribing and optimizing medications. They have found the voice of *MedStrong*—to advocate for themselves and their loved-ones and to share the message of *MedStrong* with friends and colleagues.

Many dear friends have helped with prepping for programs. Many have stood by to take pictures, to post, and to help spread the message that feeling better may come with reducing unnecessary and inappropriate medications. I thank you for your encouragement as I continue to break barriers.

Thank you to the many clients that have asked and received medication reviews and have embraced the 5-step Medication Optimization Plan (MOP). Thank you to those that have made changes through better communication with your prescribing providers. And thank you to those who have reached out to share that they feel empowered and hopeful.

Thank you to Chris Mole' for knowing that the ***MedStrong Workbook*** was a needed addition and for your design to bring the 5-Step MOP to patients and caregivers in a friendly, workable book. Thank you to Dr. Garo Safaian for your pharmacy and marketing knowledge and networking abilities. A special thank you to my podcast co-host, Dr. Kevin Walker, pharmacist and health systems specialist, in working with me and seeing the importance of pharmacy being in a pivotal role of deprescribing communications, between patients, healthcare providers, and healthcare systems. We started with *The Deprescribing Show*—and now—*The Med List* podcast. I look forward to continuing on this path and to the many future guests to interview!

Thank you to my dear WOW friend and colleague, Janet Huehls, clinical exercise physiologist. Yes, we are Women-Of-Well, sharing the message—Deprescribe to Exercise-or is it-Exercise to Deprescribe? None-the-less, we know the importance of both as we remain passionate in our fields of expertise, exploring and educating deprescribing and movement as elements of healthy aging.

Mostly, thank you to my husband, children, and hopeful future in-laws, that have provided insight, suggestions, guidance, and above all continued encouragement, love, and support.

You have all inspired me! I am truly blessed!

With love and gratitude!
~ DONNA

Contents

Introduction

HAVE YOU EVER WONDERED if you're taking too many medications and for too long? Do you ever stop to ask if they are all still necessary? Or to consider whether stopping a medication, even one you have taken for years, might make you feel better? Medications help keep us healthy and strong and can prevent or reduce the progression of chronic conditions, but they need upkeep too. Medications that have protected us, supported us, and served us well over time may need to be replaced with safer products, removed from our regimen, or reduced to lesser doses.

Being the daughter of a carpenter, I learned firsthand about the importance of building structures to last and fixing things without compromising structural soundness. But even the best-built structures need upkeep—roofs replaced, plumbing repaired, electrical panels updated. Although these elements may have served the structure well for years, changes and updates eventually become necessary for structural integrity. As a pharmacist, I take the same approach to building and updating a medication regimen, especially as my patients age.

Think of an older adult whose health you care about—a parent, grandparent, friend, partner—or maybe yourself. Do they take medications? How many? Five or more? How long have they been taking these medications? When was the last time they took something that was not prescribed, an over-the-counter remedy or supplement? Possibly every day? I have heard some patients say they take so much medication every day that they "sound like a vial of pills!"

Now think about that person's overall health. Have they been hospitalized recently? Fallen? Do they have concerns of feeling old or express issues like forgetfulness, confusion, insomnia, or weakness?

Polypharmacy, the taking of five or more prescription or nonprescription medications on a regular basis,[1] can lead to many of these conditions. It's not just the number of medications that can be harmful, but the number of unnecessary medications. Our health system is very good at prescribing medications to treat health conditions, but it's not always good at deprescribing medications that may no longer be necessary.

What is deprescribing? Deprescribing is the thoughtful process of reducing, switching, or stopping a medication that may no longer be needed or may no longer be the best treatment option. The deprescribing process should be overseen by a health-care provider in communication with the patient or a caregiver.[2] Not all medications can or should be stopped, but you may be taking medications that are no longer necessary or pose more of a risk than a benefit as you age.

Aging Changes Everything

Why is deprescribing important? Throughout the aging process, your body changes. Think of how much your body changes in your first 20, 30, or 40 years of life. Now consider how many changes a 65-year-old will experience if they live to be 85, 95, even 105. That's why considering whether a medication is still appropriate, needed, or dosed properly is an important key to healthy aging. A medication you may have started taking at 40 may not serve you well by the time you reach 80.

Your body's ability to absorb, distribute, metabolize, and eliminate medications changes throughout your lifetime, and those changes are especially acute in your older years. Changes in gut motility and acid production can change how medications are absorbed. Increased body fat and decreased hydration in older adults changes the distribution or delivery of medications throughout the body. Liver size and function decrease with age, which can reduce how well the body metabolizes medications. Age-related reduction of kidney size and function affects how well medications are eliminated from the body. Side effects may appear even after a person has taken a medication for years. Instead of taking another pill to combat the side effect, it may be possible to change, reduce, or eliminate the medication causing the ill effect.

Polypharmacy and certain medications can also lead to falls, which can be especially devastating to older adults. Though many factors contribute to falls, including health conditions, health status, sensory impairment, and environment, falls are not a "normal" part of the aging process. Deprescribing certain medications may help prevent a fall from occurring.

Do You Have Questions? You Should!

With so many factors to consider, where do you begin? How can you initiate productive conversations with health-care providers regarding the care for yourself or others? People frequently tell me, "At the pharmacy, I am asked, 'Do you have any questions?' Quite honestly, I don't know what to ask."

I understand! When my daughter was diagnosed with a brain tumor and we were waiting for more detailed tests, the medical team asked if we had any questions. My honest answer was, "Millions!" But, honestly, I could not formulate even one question at that time. Fortunately, we had the time to make a list of questions, which helped us and her medical team devise a patient-specific plan for a successful outcome.

As you read through this book, make time to develop your questions. Don't wait for a problem such as a side effect or a fall to occur. Some medications are considered potentially inappropriate or risky for older adults, so you can always start a conversation by asking a provider if you or someone you care for is taking any potentially inappropriate medications. In Part II, I will list and explain other questions you can ask.

Deprescribing is a way to optimize your medications. Stopping, reducing, or changing a medication may not have immediate results. However, over time, deprescribing may help you feel better, be more active, and maintain a better quality of life. After following a deprescribing process, some people think more clearly, have better balance, and no longer suffer from dizziness. Others feel less fatigued, stronger, and able to accomplish more every day. Others just feel better in general.

Deprescribing is different for everyone, so it is difficult to generalize how it should be done or what effects it might have. The process needs to be individualized based on a person's needs, health status or function, and health conditions.[3]

Polypharmacy is a global problem. Researchers from all over the world examine polypharmacy issues and the need to reduce prescriptions. Globally, as the number of older adults increases, experts expect the number of medications, the number of chronic diseases per individual, and problems related to polypharmacy will also rise. Building awareness of polypharmacy and taking advantage of the benefits of deprescribing can potentially reduce frailty, falls, hospitalizations, and adverse drug events. Deprescribing is a medical solution for the "condition" of polypharmacy.

You may be asking why a pharmacist or professor of pharmacy practice would write a book about reducing medications. The answer is that I want to see older adults enjoying life instead of suffering needless side effects from their medications. As a certified geriatric pharmacist, I have seen brown bags and pill boxes filled to the brim with unnecessary medications and have counseled many individuals, groups, and caregivers about medicines that need to be used with caution and prescriptions that may be more appropriate for older adults. If deprescribing can help someone feel better, move about more easily, enjoy a conversation, take a walk, or smile again, I am delighted to be part of the solution.

I do not want people to wait for the fall, the confusion, or the accident to make a change. Instead, I want to empower them to ask the right questions about their medication use so they can determine whether their medications are needed or could be changed or reduced.

After following a deprescribing process, some people think more clearly, have better balance, and no longer suffer from dizziness.

What Does This Workbook Provide?

This workbook provides the steps with examples and ample pages for your own process toward deprescribing to optimize your medications. You will learn questions to ask your health care providers, how to rethink the meds you take, and breakdown barriers that stop us from optimizing our medications. And most of all this workbook will guide you to being *MedStrong*.

To get started, think about all those involved in your health care.

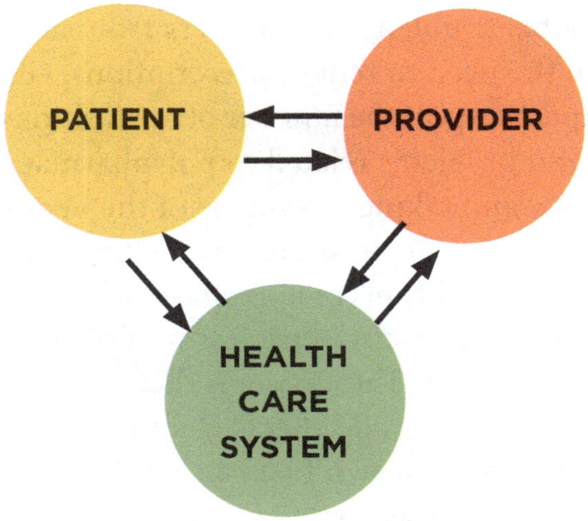

Health Care Systems

Hospital ______________________

Pharmacy ______________________

Insurance ______________________

Drug Plan ______________________

Other ______________________

____

____

____

____

Providers/Prescribers

MD ______________________

Specialists ______________________

____

____

Dentist ______________________

Optometrist ______________________

NP ______________________

PA ______________________

Other ______________________

PART I
Overmedicated

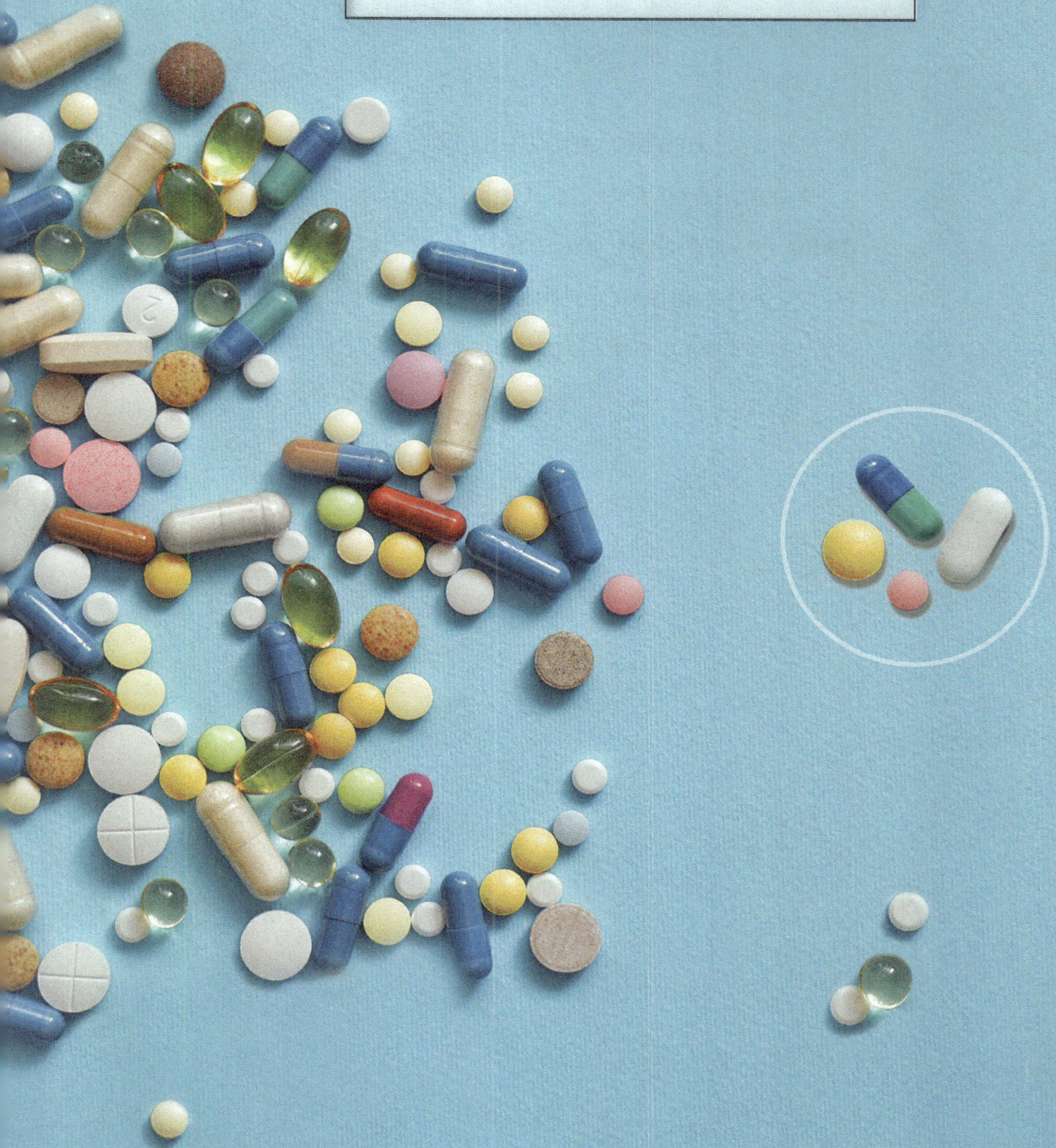

"

More significant than the number of medications you take is whether the medications being taken continue to be necessary and appropriate.

Polypharmacy

What Is Polypharmacy?

POLYPHARMACY is not necessarily defined by a particular number of medications, although the use of five or more is often used as a benchmark. But more significant than the number of medications is whether the medications being taken continue to be necessary and appropriate.[4]

Polypharmacy can be appropriate, as when someone takes several medications that are all needed, well-managed, and helpful in treating multiple chronic health conditions—for example, high blood pressure, diabetes, and asthma. Each of these conditions typically warrants multiple medications, resulting in a high number of medications prescribed.

Why Worry about Polypharmacy?

So, if polypharmacy can be appropriate and many people thrive while taking multiple medications, why should we worry about it? We need to pay attention because research has shown that polypharmacy can lead to other well-documented problems, including:

- **Prescribing cascades**
- **Overuse, underuse, or misuse of medications**
- **Complex regimens with questionable benefits**
- **Increased risk of frailty and hospital admissions**
- **Greater experiences of geriatric syndromes**
- **Higher risks of adverse drug events, including drug interactions**

Let's take a closer look at some of these potential problems.

Polypharmacy can lead to prescribing cascades

A prescribing cascade is where one medication can lead to another. Because more side effects can occur when a patient takes more medications, even more medications may be prescribed to treat these adverse effects. The opposite is also true: a prescribing cascade can lead to polypharmacy when "unnecessary" medications are added to treat a side effect instead of changing the original medication to avoid the side effect.

As you can see, it is easy to wind up in a polypharmacy situation. To avoid prescribing cascades, be sure you know exactly why you take each of your medications and why your provider thinks each is necessary for you. Becoming an educated health consumer can help you keep your medications in check.

IN REAL LIFE

The following scenario illustrates how prescribing cascades may sometimes be necessary initially but continued needlessly—and possibly to a harmful effect.

Diuretics (sometimes called "water pills") have for many years been a first-line medication against high blood pressure. But some prescribed diuretics can reduce potassium, so health-care providers subsequently add a prescription for supplemental potassium. This diuretic-plus-potassium combination is considered a prescribing cascade because the diuretic lowers potassium levels, causing the patient to take another medication to counteract or correct the effect of the original medication. The combination can be very effective if managed well but can become problematic if it is not.

Mr. K, an older gentleman, had taken the diuretic, hydrochlorothiazide (HCTZ), for approximately 25 years to reduce blood pressure. He was also taking potassium chloride to keep his potassium levels normal and was prescribed other medication as he grew older. When Mr. K lost weight and began experiencing orthostatic hypotension, or low blood pressure, when he stood up, it was decided that the diuretic was no longer necessary because his blood pressure was within normal range. Deprescribing HCTZ would potentially reduce the risk of orthostatic hypotension.

But when it came time for his next 90-day refills, Mr. K called in for a refill of his potassium tablets. The pharmacist asked if he still needed the HCTZ but was told that medication had been stopped by the doctor. Recognizing that the potassium tablets were probably no longer necessary if the HCTZ had been stopped, the pharmacist checked with the physician, who confirmed that the HCTZ was indeed deprescribed and then stated, "Oh yeah, the potassium can also be discontinued."

Had the potassium not been stopped, Mr. K's potassium levels would have increased over time and a potential abnormal heart rhythm could have occurred, resulting in hospitalization.

Polypharmacy can cause overuse, underuse, or misuse of medications and can result in complex regimens with questionable benefits. [5]

Overuse can occur when someone is confused or forgetful, which can lead them to forget they have taken a medication and then take it again. My mother would help my grandfather manage his medications by placing his medicines in a pill organizer. Later in the week, she would discover that medications were missing from many days in addition to the ones that were supposed to be taken.

Underuse can follow the same scenario. Perhaps you can't remember if you've taken a particular prescription today, so you just decide not to take it. Maybe you just forget about one of your medications. This can happen especially with medicines that are supposed to be taken multiple times per day.

Misuse of medication can happen because of confusion about the correct dose or the timing of the medication. Or you might misunderstand specific instructions or confuse one medication for another. I once counseled an older adult about her intake of daily aspirin. Her doctor told her to "take baby aspirin every day," so the woman went to the pharmacy, bought baby aspirin, and took four baby aspirin, four times daily, as instructed on the box. However, those instructions are for pain and fever relief.

When I reviewed her medication, I explained that her doctor wanted her to take aspirin for heart protection, so probably wanted her to take only one tablet, once a day. I asked if she had any bruising, if her gums bled easily when she brushed or flossed, or if she had nose bleeds. She had not experienced any of those side effects but was very embarrassed by her misuse of the aspirin. I explained that she had done what she was told, which was to "take aspirin daily." Because she was not given specific instructions, she followed the directions on the box, leading to misuse of a medication that could have led to harmful effects.

Complex regimens can occur from complicated medication directions that make it hard for some users to understand or follow all the directions. For example, some medications need to be taken regularly—sometimes multiple times a day—while other medications are used only for flare-ups of the same condition. Individuals need to know when to take certain medications and not confuse a rescue medication with a maintenance medication. The more prescriptions a user has, the easier it is to get confused about the necessary regimen.

Questions about the *benefits* of multiple medications also grow as more medications are added, because more medications can lead to more side effects and more adverse events. More medications also increase the risk of additive effects and interactions.

Polypharmacy increases the risk of adverse events, including drug interactions.

Drug interactions can be drug–drug, drug–disease, drug–food, or drug–alcohol interactions.

Drug-drug interactions occur when a combination of drugs causes one or more of the meds to work differently in a person's body. There may be an increased effect, a decreased effect, or an additive effect.

Increased effects typically occur when one medication causes another medication to have a higher exposure to the receptors in the body, which may lead to more side effects or toxicities. For example, amlodipine, a common blood pressure medication, can cause simvastatin, a common cholesterol-lowering medication, to have more exposure or availability, which could cause users to experience muscle aches and pains from the higher amounts of simvastatin available in the body.

Decreased effects occur when combining medications causes one or more of the drugs to be less effective. Tamoxifen is a medication used for breast cancer patients to reduce the risk of the cancer returning. If the antidepressant fluoxetine, for example, is also taken, then the tamoxifen is less likely to be effective because fluoxetine interferes with its activity. This interaction could result in tamoxifen being ineffective and potentially result in a return of the breast cancer.

An additive type of drug interaction happens when multiple medications are combined and produce similar outcomes or side effects. For example, more than one drug may be used to reduce blood pressure, or several antibiotics may be combined to treat a complicated infection. These combination therapies are not necessarily harmful and, in fact, may have a beneficial effect. When multiple medications have similar side effects, however, such as drowsiness or dizziness, the combination of drugs can cause an additive effect that could be harmful.

Drug-disease interactions occur when a medication being used to treat one condition makes another condition worse. For example, many OTC medication labels state, "Do not take if" or "Consult your doctor or pharmacist if" you have certain conditions. For example, a decongestant for cold or allergy could increase blood pressure, worsening existing hypertension. Pain relief medications, such as ibuprofen or naproxen, may worsen types of heart disease, including heart failure. It is important to heed the warnings on OTC labels so you do not worsen other conditions while self-treating for a different problem. It is just as important to read the prescription information sheets you receive from the pharmacy to be certain that your prescribed medications will not worsen other conditions.

Drug-food interactions are typically noted on prescription drugs with auxiliary label cautions—the used-to-be colorful stickers and now yellow precaution stickers—that may be added to your prescription label. Prescriptions with labels warning about the intake of dairy or grapefruit are common. Many prescriptions instruct users to allow for a two-hour window of separation between dairy consumption and drug intake. That's because dairy products contain calcium, which can reduce the absorption of certain medications, causing a reduced benefit.

Warnings about eating grapefruit are typically placed on cholesterol-lowering agents known as statins. When combined with grapefruit, many statins are not metabolized properly and can accumulate in the body, causing a "stacking," dose by dose, to high levels that may cause side effects, especially muscle pain and weakness. (Note: Not all statins are affected by grapefruit; for example, grapefruit can be enjoyed without worry when one is taking rosuvastatin or pravastatin. If you love grapefruit, asking your health-care provider something as simple as, "Can I eat grapefruit with this?" can allow for a better match between you and your prescription.)

Alcohol affects all systems of the body; therefore, it is no surprise that several medications—prescription and OTC—can cause ***drug–alcohol interactions.*** On its own, alcohol can cause confusion, upset stomach, stomach bleeds, seizures, blurred vision, increased heart rate, low heart rate, arrhythmias, dry mouth, unsteadiness, stumbling, falls, insomnia, sleepiness, and more. As with medications, alcohol is less easily tolerated, causes more side effects, and is more difficult to metabolize and eliminate as we age. Many medications cause side effects similar to those caused by alcohol, so taking any of those medications with alcohol can lead to additive effects and more severe reactions. The National Institutes of Health offer a booklet online that provides drug–alcohol interaction information.[6]

Polypharmacy and unnecessary medications may lead to geriatric syndromes

We like to blame many ailments on advancing age, including constipation, cognition deficits, falls, hospitalizations, uncontrolled bladder, weight loss, dizziness, blood pressure changes, unsteadiness, arrhythmias, mood changes, and other issues that negatively affect quality of life. But many of these "age-related" conditions may actually be caused or worsened by polypharmacy or unnecessary medications. Many medications are directly associated with these conditions, which may resolve if a medication is reduced, changed, or stopped. The form on page 9 lists some types of medications that may contribute to age-related conditions or geriatric syndromes.[7]

Check Your Concerns About the Medications You Take

- ☐ **Prescribing cascades** ______________________
- ☐ **Overuse** ______________________
- ☐ **Underuse** ______________________
- ☐ **Misuse** ______________________
- ☐ **Complex regimen** ______________________
- ☐ **Hospitalizations** ______________________
- ☐ **The way I feel could be my meds and not my age** ______________________
- ☐ **Drug-Drug interactions** ______________________
- ☐ **Drug-Disease interactions** ______________________
- ☐ **Drug-food Interactions** ______________________
- ☐ **Drug-alcohol interactions** ______________________
- ☐ **Becoming frail** ______________________

Medications and Age-Related Conditions

On the next page, check or highlight the geriatric syndrome you experience and if you take any of the types of medications associated with the syndrome.

Note: This is not an exhaustive list. If you experience a particular geriatric syndrome, speak with your health care providers / advocate. If you take a particular type of medication you may not be experiencing the geriatric syndrome currently, but it is a good idea to think about the potential of the adverse effect and be proactive about the benefit versus the harm of the medication as you age.

We love to blame age for many "conditions" though it may be medications that are causing the issues.

Medications That May Contribute to Age-Related Conditions

Geriatric Syndrome	Types of Medications
☐ **Delirium** ☐ **Dementia** ☐ **Cognitive deficit** ☐ **Confusion**	☐ Medications for overactive bladder ☐ Antidepressants ☐ Medications for allergies ☐ Antipsychotics ☐ Medications for stomach spasms ☐ Muscle relaxants ☐ Benzodiazepines / medications for anxiety/insomnia ☐ Corticosteroids
☐ **Falls**	☐ Medications used for seizures ☐ Medications to control high blood pressure ☐ Antipsychotics ☐ Medications used for insomnia ☐ Benzodiazepines & medications for anxiety and insomnia, incl. TCAs (e.g., amitriptyline) and SSRIs (e.g., paroxetine)
☐ **Overactive bladder**	☐ Medications used for Alzheimer's ☐ Diuretics ("water pills")
☐ **Dizziness** ☐ **Drop in blood pressure**	☐ Medications for overactive bladder ☐ Medications for high blood pressure ☐ Medications for diabetes such as glyburide and glipizide ☐ Antidepressants ☐ Medications for allergies ☐ Antipsychotics ☐ Opioids for pain relief ☐ Medications for insomnia
☐ **Difficulty swallowing**	☐ Medications to strengthen bones ☐ NSAIDs (e.g., ibuprofen, naproxen) ☐ Potassium
☐ **Taste/smell aversion**	☐ Blood pressure meds ☐ Antibiotics ☐ Medications for allergies ☐ Eye drops
☐ **Reduced appetite**	☐ Antibiotics ☐ Medications for seizures ☐ Digoxin ☐ Benzodiazepines ☐ Metformin ☐ Opioids ☐ Antidepressants
☐ **Constipation**	☐ Overactive bladder medications ☐ allergy medications ☐ Opioids ☐ Calcium channel blockers, (e.g., verapamil) ☐ Iron

How Does Polypharmacy Occur?

In an article called "Easy to Start, Hard to Stop," which focuses on polypharmacy and deprescribing, Dr. Barbara Farrell shares a common scenario that demonstrates how easily polypharmacy can occur.[8]

> *A medication is started to see how it will help, possibly even as a diagnostic trial, then the medication is continued. Ten years then go by and the primary care doctor retires. The patient sees a new primary care physician who is not quite certain why a patient is on a particular medication but is uneasy about stopping the medication. Now the patient is in their 80s and has been on the medication for 30 years, yet no one really knows why.*

This is a common scenario, where the patient is not having difficulties at the time of the appointment, and all seems well and good.

What Medications Have You Taken for 10 or More Years?

Medication	Number of Years

How Willing are You to Make a Change to Your Medications?

On a scale of 1-10, circle how likely are you willing stop, reduce, or change a medication you take?

(unlikely) < 1 2 3 4 5 6 7 8 9 10 > (very likely)

Are you resistant to stop certain medications?
List any medications you are fearful of stopping and why?

____

____

____

____

____

____

Do you feel overwhelmed by change? If so, jot down why that is.

____

____

____

____

____

Polypharmacy may slow decision-making abilities, reduce cognitive processing, and contribute to reluctance to make changes.

- **ASK FOR HELP** if you are overwhelmed
- **IDENTIFY** what is overwhelming.
- **SPEAKING ABOUT YOUR CONCERNS** with a health care advocate may help the process to be less overwhelming.

The Ever-Changing Body

YOUR BODY CHANGES THROUGHOUT YOUR LIFETIME. It's easier to understand this concept when you think about pediatric patients. You would typically not give the same dose of a medication to a one-year-old as you would to an 18-year-old. Although adults' bodies may not outwardly change as drastically as children's bodies, changes in absorption, distribution, metabolism, and elimination (ADME) occur throughout the aging process. Thus, the medication dose you take at age 40 may not be the appropriate dose for you at 70, even if you are still roughly the same height and weight and even though prescribing guidelines are often the same for adults, regardless of age.

ADME

ADME stands for the absorption, distribution, metabolism, and elimination of a medication; in other words, what happens when we take a medication.

Absorption
Describes how a drug finds its way to our blood- stream and receptors. For oral medications it involves the gut—otherwise known as the gastrointestinal tract.

Distribution
Describes where the drug goes in the body: the brain, the blood, muscle. Blood flow, water/fluid volume, fat, and proteins all affect the body's distribution of a medication.

Metabolism
Describes how medication changes in the body. Some changes may activate a medication or prepare it to be eliminated from the body, a process that relies on liver function.

Elimination
Describes the excretion of the drug from the body, which typically relies on kidney and bowel function.

Consider how your body has changed throughout the years.
For better or worse the body is ever-changing.

____

____

____

____

____

How Aging Can Change ADME

Absorption can be affected by gut health and medications, such as proton pump inhibitors that reduce acid levels in the stomach. As you age, your gut functions slow, and medications may not be as readily absorbed. Slower absorption rates may be more problematic for acute or quick-acting medications, such as pain-relievers or antibiotics that need to be absorbed for appropriate therapeutic and beneficial levels.

Slower absorption may not cause as many problems with medications taken for chronic conditions because these types of medications are monitored for a particular outcome. Doses can be raised or lowered, depending upon clinical (how you are feeling) and therapeutic (how your labs and vitals are responding to the medication) outcomes.

Distribution also changes over time. Most people tend to have more body fat later in life, and more fat means medications that are fat-loving—lipophilic—may remain in the body longer before they are eliminated. In addition, aging can lead to decreased thirst perception, lessened fluid intake, and higher likelihood of dehydration. Medications that are water-loving—hydrophilic—tend to accumulate in the body at higher concentrations when there is less hydration and more dehydration. In both cases, more fat or less hydration, lower doses of medications may be needed to prevent increased side effects and toxicity.

Metabolism changes in an aging body due to smaller liver size, less blood flow to the liver, and poor liver function. A slowing metabolism reduces the ability of the body to convert a drug to a product ready for elimination, leading to more side effects and toxicity of the medication. Conversely, some medications need to be metabolized to an active form to be helpful; when this process is reduced, then the effectiveness of the medication is also reduced. To make things even more challenging, older adults are likely to be taking multiple medications that are competing to be metabolized.

Elimination of medications typically occurs through the kidneys. Like the liver, kidneys also decrease in size, have less blood flow, and may not function as well as people age. If drugs and the byproducts of metabolism are not eliminated, then medication concentrations can increase, causing side effects and toxicity. Kidney function can be calculated for proper dosing and management of medications, and the equation used to determine kidney function includes age as a factor. Age inversely affects kidney function: the higher the age, the lower the kidney function.

A CLOSER LOOK: Pharmacokinetics and Pharmacodynamics

ADME (absorption, distribution, metabolism, and elimination) are the components of pharmacokinetics: what the body does to the drug, when a medication will begin to work, how long its peak will last, its half-life for elimination purposes, and how the drug is eliminated. These functions or kinetics can be altered with age.

Another factor is pharmacodynamics: what the drug does to the body. Aging individuals can become more susceptible and sensitive to side effects such as lightheadedness, confusion, fatigue, constipation, cardiovascular effects, and dry mouth. The central nervous system may be more easily affected in older adults because of changes in the blood-brain barrier and increased side effects of medications. Even if you have taken a medication for years, your body changes as you age and may react differently.

I have felt the following effects: *(Check the boxes that apply.)*

- ☐ **Lightheaded** ________________
- ☐ **Confused** ________________
- ☐ **Fatigued** ________________
- ☐ **Constipated** ________________
- ☐ **Heart palpitations** ________________
- ☐ **Dry mouth** ________________
- ☐ **Other:** *List how you feel: stomach upset, headaches, achy, weak, etc.*

____

____

► **ASK: COULD MY MEDS BE CAUSING THESE?**

Or maybe you feel GREAT! We want you to feel that way!

Deprescribing is best when it is a proactive approach!

Don't wait for the fall, hospitalization, or accident to occur.

Potentially Inappropriate Medications

Inappropriate medications will vary from person to person. Here are some ideas to consider if a medication may be inappropriate. Jot down medications you may want to question.

1. Medication is still being used even though a health condition has resolved.

Ex: Acid reflux is resolved but medication (omeprazole) is continued.

____

____

____

____

____

2. Medication or combination of medications are continued beyond the needed time frame.

Ex: Anticoagulant and aspirin are continued beyond recommended time frame after cardiovascular stents are placed.

____

____

____

____

____

3. Medication is continued or increased despite questionable benefit.

Ex: Gabapentin used for pain, yet pain not resolved.

____

____

____

____

4. A non-prescription medication is being used with a prescription medication for the same issue.

Ex: Fish oil and statins.

5. Medications are being taken that counteract benefits of each.

Ex: Donepezil used for dementia causes incontinence. Oxybutynin used for incontinence causes dementia.

6. Medications dosed too aggressively.

Ex: Blood pressure medications causing lightheadedness.

Analysis of Polypharmacy

Number of medications you take: ____________

Which medications did you find concerning during this process?

Medication: ____________________

Concern: ____________________

____

____

Medication: ____________________

Concern: ____________________

____

____

Medication: ____________________

Concern: ____________________

____

____

Medication: ____________________

Concern: ____________________

____

____

Medication: ____________________

Concern: ____________________

____

Medication: ____________________

Concern: ____________________

____

Medication Quality and Quality of Life

Now that you have explored the idea of polypharmacy, you can look at the quality of the medications—prescription and non-prescription—that you take. Perhaps some of the complications of polypharmacy or how you feel may have caused you to question some of your meds.

In Part II: What Can We DO?, we will begin the work of the deprescribing process using the Medication Optimization Plan (MOP).

OVERVIEW OF PART I: Overmedicated

- Polypharmacy can be appropriate and beneficial, but it can become an inappropriate and unhelpful overload of medications.
- Medication overload can occur from prescription medications that were never necessary, medications that do not benefit the patient, unnecessary OTC medications, or medications that were once necessary but are no longer needed.
- The more medications a person takes, the higher the risk of an adverse drug event.
- Even "mild" adverse effects, such as dizziness, lightheadedness, nausea, or incontinence, can affect a person's quality of daily living. More severe adverse effects, including delirium, cognitive changes, falls, and bleeding, may lead to life-threatening scenarios and possibly death.
- The culture to prescribe, patient expectations about the benefits of medications, direct-to-consumer advertisements, and marketing to prescribers add to the polypharmacy fire.
- Lifestyle changes may be more beneficial and allow for better quality of life than a full pill box. Multiple medications should not be considered the norm.

PART II

What Can We DO? Deprescribe to Optimize

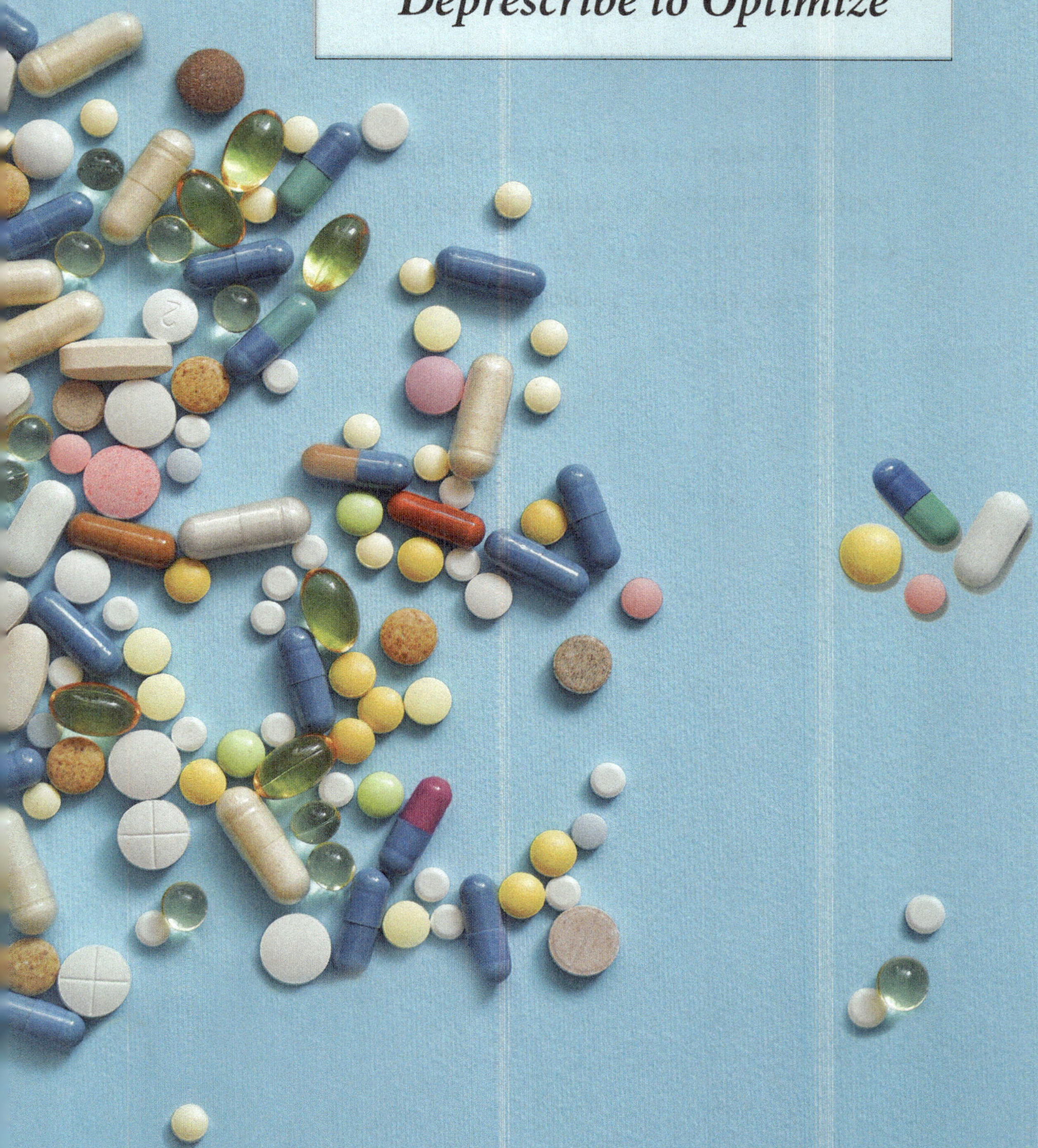

“

The process of deprescribing is just as valuable to quality health-care practices as is the process of prescribing medications.

REMEDY:
REthink the MEDs You Take

DEPRESCRIBING IS A PATH TO OPTIMIZING medications for the individual. It should be a thoughtful process to identify medications that may have more risk than benefit or that may no longer fit the individual's healthcare needs or goals. The process of deprescribing is just as valuable to quality health-care practices as is the process of prescribing medications.

What is Deprescribing?

When deprescribing, patients or caregivers work with their health-care providers to determine whether a medication may be causing more harm than good and whether that medication can be reduced, changed, or stopped. The patient is monitored and followed after the change, just as when a new medication is started.[9] Deprescribing is a positive, active approach to "patient-centered care" that can help improve health outcomes and reduce adverse drug reactions; enhancing a patient's quality of life.

Are Prescribing and Deprescribing Similar?

The concept of deprescribing is taking on new significance. Advancements in medical treatments allow people to live longer with multiple medical conditions, which may lead to multiple medications. A component of good prescribing is deprescribing, but our healthcare culture is geared more toward starting medications rather than ending them, which can lead to polypharmacy and its associated challenges, which were discussed in Part I. Prescribers are inclined to initiate treatment, and patients are often willing to add and continue medications but less supportive of decreasing treatment. Eventually, medication becomes a burden instead of offering beneficial outcomes.[10]

Adding and Subtracting Medication

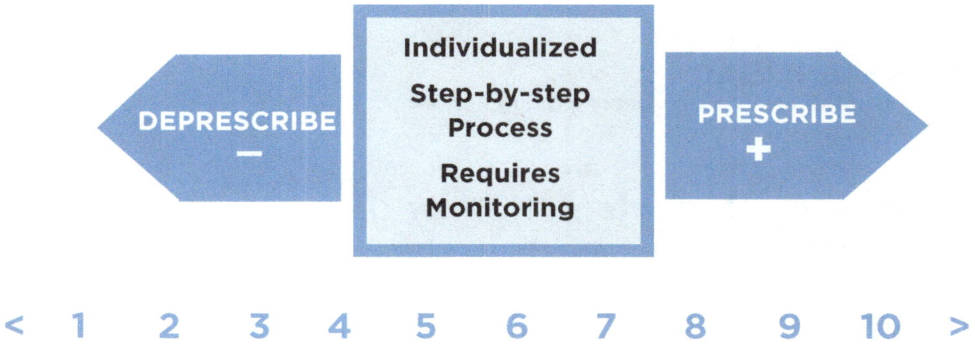

Why Deprescribe?

Evidence of the benefits of deprescribing is growing with many medications that could become inappropriate or may be inappropriate from the outset.[11] Deprescribing antihypertensives (blood pressure medication), antipsychotics (for psychosis and agitation in older adults with dementia), and benzodiazepines (for sleep and anxiety) has been reported to reduce patient falls and cardiovascular events and improve cognition and motor function without adverse effects.[12, 13, 14, 15]

Deprescribing can also lead to cost containment for individuals, the older adult care community, and the health-care system. Because fewer prescriptions may lead to lower costs and fewer adverse events, falls, and accidents, many individuals and organizations may reap financial benefits of deprescribing practices.

Where to Begin: Medication Optimization Plan

So, now that you know the risks of polypharmacy and the benefits of deprescribing, what should you do next? How do you start the process? And how do you know whether a particular medication should be deprescribed, especially if you do not have a background or expertise in pharmacology or medicine? Use the following method.

MedStrong Medication Optimization Plan (MOP)
Step-by-Step Deprescribing Guide for the Patient

STEP 1 — **List all Medications.**
Fill out the MedStrong Medication List.

STEP 2 — **Review Medication List.**
Use the MedStrong Medication List and the MedStrong Question List to formulate questions.

STEP 3 — **Decide to Deprescribe with Your Provider.**
Start the "DO" conversation using the Medstrong Question List.

STEP 4 — **Make a Plan.**
Fill out the MedStrong Deprescribing Form.

STEP 5 — **Monitor, Document, Follow-up.**
Use the Medstrong Deprescribing Form and the MedStrong Medication Change Form.

STEP 1 **List all Medications.**
Fill out the MedStrong Medication List.

List ALL Your Prescriptions

Fill out the MedStrong Medication List

Be certain to include:

- tablets
- capsules
- liquids
- powders
- injectables
- eye drops
- ear drops
- nasal sprays
- inhalers
- creams
- nebulizers
- as needed products

MedStrong PRESCRIPTION Medication List

PRESCRIPTION Name of Prescription Medication and Strength of Dose	How Taken	Reason for Taking	Does the Problem Still Exist?	Is the Medical Condition Controlled?
1.				
2.				
3.				
4.				
5.				
6.				
7.				
8.				
9.				
10.				
11.				
12.				
13.				
14.				
15.				

List ALL Your Non-Prescription Medications

Fill out the MedStrong OTC Medication List

Be certain to include:

- vitamins
- creams
- supplements
- eye drops
- herbals
- self-treatment as needed meds

MedStrong OVER-THE-COUNTER Medication List

OVER THE COUNTER OTC Medication, Supplement, or Herbal and Strength of Dose	How Taken	Reason for Taking	Does the Problem Still Exist?	Is the Medical Condition Controlled?
1.				
2.				
3.				
4.				
5.				
6.				
7.				
8.				
9.				
10.				
11.				
12.				
13.				
14.				
15.				
16.				
17.				

STEP 2

Review Medication List.

Use the MedStrong Medication List and the MedStrong Question List to formulate questions.

Prescription Medications

- Look at the Medication List you just made. Are there question marks? Uncertainties?
- Formulate questions around these unknowns. List your questions here:

PRESCRIPTION MEDICATION	Question

Over the Counter Medications

- Are you taking OTCs, supplements, vitamins, herbals?
- What are you trying to treat?
- What are you hoping to alleviate or how are you thinking you benefit from the product?

NON-PRESCRIPTIONS	Purpose	Question

MedStrong QUESTION LIST

Check the questions, to ask your health-care providers, that fit your concerns.

Questions to Ask Yourself

- ☐ Am I having problems paying for all of my prescriptions?
- ☐ Do I sometimes choose which medicines to take or not take because of affordability issues?
- ☐ Do I take some or all of my medications differently than how they were prescribed to "stretch them out"? For example, do I take a pill every other day even if it is prescribed to take daily?

Questions to Ask Your Health-Care Provider

- ☐ Are there any medications that I am currently taking that may no longer be necessary?
- ☐ Are there any medications that may be dosed too high for my age, health status, kidney function, or with other medications I am taking?
- ☐ Could one of my health concerns actually be a side effect of a medication?
- ☐ Are there safer medications I could be taking?
- ☐ Can any of my medications increase my risk of falls?
- ☐ Can any combination of these medications increase my risk of falls or increase a risk of bleeding?

Questions to Ask at the Pharmacy

- ☐ Could I be using an OTC product to treat a side effect of one of my prescription medications?
- ☐ Is this OTC product okay to take with my current medications and my health conditions?
- ☐ Are any of my medications potentially being prescribed for a side effect of another prescription (prescribing cascade)?
- ☐ Could any of my medications increase my risk of falling? If so, which ones?
- ☐ If I could take fewer medications, which ones should I ask my doctor about possibly stopping?
- ☐ Am I taking any unnecessary medications?
- ☐ How long will it take for this medication to start working as it should?
- ☐ Is this a medication that I need to fill regularly?
- ☐ When would be the best time of day to take this medication?
- ☐ Is it possible for you to help me figure out a schedule to take my medications?

Questions to Ask When an Older Adult Is Hospitalized

- ☐ Could any of my medications—prescription, OTC, herbal, or supplements—have contributed to this condition?
- ☐ Could my medications have interacted to have caused my hospitalization, such as medications that have additive effects / side effects?
- ☐ Are there any of my current medications that might be unnecessary or that you think we should discuss with the primary care physician or specialist?
- ☐ Are there any medications, OTCs, or supplements that may be interacting with blood tests or any other tests or procedures?

____

____

____

Questions to Ask When Being Discharged from the Hospital

- ☐ Are there changes to my medications or how I should take them?
- ☐ Are there medications that are similar to medications that I take at home? I do not want to duplicate my medications.
- ☐ Are there any medications I should no longer take?
- ☐ How long should I continue taking any new medications?

Are some just for a short period of time or just when needed?

____

____

My Questions about Specific Concerns or Specific Medications

____

Each area of health care is a possible setting to ask about your medications:

- At the Pharmacy
- At the MD's Office
- At the Specialist
- At the Hospital
- At the NP and PA Office
- At the Short-term Rehab
- At the Long-term Care Facility
- At the Dentist
- At the Optometrist
- At the Physical Therapist
- At the Occupational Therapist
- With Hospice or Palliative Care Team

More Conversation Starters

You've come up with several ideas in the past few pages about how to start deprescribing conversations in certain settings. Here are a few more ideas, which have been adapted from an article in the *American Family Physician.*[16] These guidelines were originally written to help health-care providers open conversations about deprescribing. But they have been adapted here to help show patients how to open conversations with their physicians.

Exploring options

- How important is it that I take [name your medication]?
- It is important to me that I continue to take medications I need, but I would be willing to stop some medications if I could.
- Can we decide if I really need to take all these medications?
- I would like to try a trial of stopping or reducing [name the medication] to see how it goes.
- If the medication(s) could be causing side effects, could we try to stop or reduce it/them to see if it helps?

Benefit versus risk

- If we decide to reduce or stop [name your medication], how might I feel? How will I know whether I am benefitting from the change or if I need to restart the medicine?
- I am taking several medications now. I would like to review these regularly to be sure that each one is still a benefit and to check for side effects.
- I understand that medication side effects can add up. Do my medications have some similar side effects that could be making me tired, constipated, forgetful, fall? [Fill in your specific condition here.]
- I read that as we age, medications we have taken successfully for years may become more of a harm than a benefit and no longer needed. Are some medications I take a concern? I'm wondering about [mention any meds you have taken for a long period of time].
- I heard some medications are needed only for a short period of time, but it seems like I have been taking [name your medication] for quite some time.

Talking Deprescribing with your Loved Ones

Caregivers can sometimes talk directly to health-care providers about deprescribing, but they usually have to first broach the topic directly with their loved one. How do family members or caregivers bring up deprescribing when they fear their loved one will be resistant to the idea?

- Explain that deprescribing is a thoughtful process and a way to optimize their medications.
- Explain that the change does not have to be set in stone. The patient will be monitored to see how they feel when medications are reduced, switched, or stopped.
- Celebrate them for being proactive in their health.
- Take a positive approach that you want them to stay healthy or feel better.

STEP 3

Decide to Deprescribe with Your Provider.

Start the "DO" conversation using the Medstrong Question List.

Let's have a conversation! And take notes or have someone take notes for you.

Primary Care

Specialist

Hospital Setting

Long-Term Care

Shared Decision-Making

If you are uncertain what to do regarding your medications or you have a choice:

- **ASK: What would you do if you were me? (This is an acceptable question, but it does not need to be the ultimate decision.)**
- **List the pros and cons to help you decide.**

Medication ____________________

PROS	CONS

Medication ____________________

PROS	CONS

Medication ____________________

PROS	CONS

STEP 4 Make a Plan.

Fill out the MedStrong Deprescribing Form.

Fill out the ***MedStrong Deprescribing Form***

- It's important to write things down
- Many meds look alike and sound a like
- Taking notes can reduce being overwhelmed with trying to recall information
- Good practices include writing things down
- Repeat instructions to double-check that you have it right

► **ASK: Just so I have the correct information,** let me repeat what you told me (then repeat what you think is correct or what you need to do).

Fill out the top half of ***MedStrong Deprescribing Form*** for each medication that you plan to deprescribe (the second half is the monitoring and follow-up).

MedStrong Deprescribing Form

Medication: ______________________ **Date:** ______________

Why is this medication being deprescribed? ______________________

DEPRESCRIBE INSTRUCTIONS:

Changed to: ________ **Reduced to:** ________ **Stopped: Date:** ________

Taper: ☐ **Yes** ☐ **No** **If yes, taper instructions:** ______________

MONITOR:

Labs: ______________ Date: ______________

Check: ______________ and keep a log.

(Examples: blood pressure, heart rate, blood glucose, weight)

Date: Time: Results:

HOW DO I FEEL?:

☐ No different: ______________________

☐ Not so good because: ______________________

☐ Better, I notice that: ______________________

FOLLOW-UP WITH:

Name of health care provider: ______________________

Phone number: ______________________

Date of next appointment: ______________________

STEP 5 Monitor, Document, Follow-up.

Use the Medstrong Deprescribing Form and the MedStrong Medication Change Form.

Use the ***MedStrong Deprescribing Form*** and ***MedStrong Medication Change Form.*** This final step is important, monitor the changes in your health and body and record the relevant information on the ***MedStrong Deprescribing Form***. Monitoring and follow-up help close the loop on the deprescribing process to ensure that the changes are helpful and not harmful.

- Will you need to check lab results in order to monitor your health conditions after you stop or change a particular medication? Record that here.
- Do you need to keep an eye on a vital sign and log the results for your follow-up appointment? Record that here.

MedStrong Deprescribing Form

Medication: ______________________ Date: ______________

Why is this medication being deprescribed? ______________________

DEPRESCRIBE INSTRUCTIONS:

Changed to: __________ Reduced to: __________ Stopped: Date: __________

Taper: ☐ Yes ☐ No If yes, taper instructions: ______________________

MONITOR:

Labs: ______________________ **Date:** ______________________

Check: ______________________ **and keep a log.**

(Examples: blood pressure, heart rate, blood glucose, weight)

Date:__________ **Time:** __________ **Results:** ______________

HOW DO I FEEL?:

☐ **No different:** ______________________

☐ **Not so good because:** ______________________

☐ **Better, I notice that:** ______________________

FOLLOW-UP WITH:

Name of health care provider:______________________

Phone number:______________________

Date of next appointment:______________________

NOTE: "No Change" to how you feel can be a perfectly GOOD outcome!

Medication Change Form

Checklist after knowing that the med is no longer necessary:

- ☐ Document the change!
- ☐ Stop auto-refills.
- ☐ Stop mail-order of the medications.
- ☐ Dispose of medications correctly.
- ☐ Update your medication list too!!!

MedStrong Medication Change Form

Medication and Strength	How Many, How Often	Prescribed by	Date/ Year Started	Still Taking?	Date Medication Stopped or Changed	Medication Restarted or Changed, Why?

Deprescribing Dynamics

The intertwinings of polypharmacy and deprescribing is illustrated in the ***Deprescribing —Polypharmacy Diagram*** below. As depicted, polypharmacy can increase anticholinergic burden and frailty. Anticholinergic burden can increase frailty. Being proactive with deprescribing can reduce all three factors:

- The number of medications
- Unwanted side effects
- Worsening frailty

Deprescribing-Polypharmacy Diagram

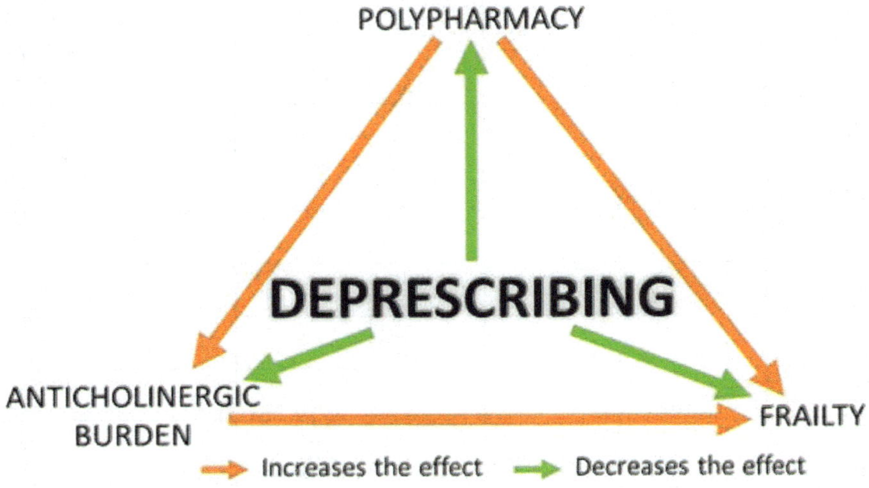

In the next section you will learn more about medications that may be worth evaluating for continued need and if a med is still a benefit. Remember, something that is beneficial now may not be a couple years from now.

Keep asking! Make deprescribing conversations a part of your health checks.

> ▶ **THINK ABOUT IT**
>
> **Isn't it worth the time and effort to rethink your meds?**

What's in Your Pill Box?

THE FIRST STEP IN THE *MedStrong Medication Optimization Plan (MOP)* is to list all your medications. As you continue through the process of formulating questions, discussing your medications with your providers, and eventually working through the deprescribe to optimize (DO) steps, certain types of medications should get priority attention, especially if they are being taken by an older adult. These types of medications include antipsychotics, statins, antihypertensives, benzodiazepines, proton pump inhibitors (PPIs), anticholinergics, sedatives, opioids, and nonsteroidal anti-inflammatory drugs (NSAIDs), including aspirin and COX-2 inhibitors, such as celecoxib.

Anticholinergics ("anti-coal-in-er-jix")

Anticholinergic medications are used for Parkinson's, urinary incontinence, overactive bladder, stomach spasms, nausea, vomiting, and chronic obstructive pulmonary disease (COPD). Many additional medications, including muscle relaxants, older first-generation antihistamines (used for allergies and sleep), medications used for depression and anxiety, and antipsychotics also have anticholinergic properties or side effects.

Anticholinergics should be prime suspects in a search for potentially inappropriate medications. They can be very drying, causing dry eyes, dry nasal passages, dry mouth, difficulty swallowing, and urinary retention—that's why they are frequently used as incontinence medications. Other side effects include fast heart rate, confusion, and balance issues that can increase the risk of falls.

Anticholinergics used for	
urinary incontinence	oxybutynin, solifenacin, tolterodine
COPD	aclidinium, ipratropium, tiotropium, umeclidinium
parkinsonism	benztropine
stomach spasm	dicyclomine, hyoscyamine
motion sickness, nausea, vomiting	scopolamine

MedStrong Anticholinergic Burden Scoring Sheet

Date:____________________ Scale Used: ______________________________

Medication	Listed on anticholinergic scale? Y/N	Score
	Number of medications Y =	Total:

► ASK: What is my anticholinergic burden?

- **If its 3 or more consider asking to reduce your anticholinergic burden.**
- **Especially if you experience: dry eyes, dry mouth, constipation, confusion, fatigue, grogginess, unsteadiness, fast heart rate, and falls.**
- **Anticholinergic Burden Calculator: Calculate your anticholinergic burden online at http://www.acbcalc.com**

Antipsychotics

Antipsychotics are medications used to treat delirium, disorientation, paranoia, schizophrenia, and bipolar disorders. These medications can be used short-term (episodically) or long-term.

Quetiapine and aripiprazole are FDA-approved for bipolar disorder and schizophrenia, but they are also commonly used as an off-label therapy in older adults for agitation associated with dementia.

Quetiapine is also frequently seen on medication lists to be taken in the evening to improve sleep. Many products are used in this type of off-label fashion, but these medications, due to their potential side effects, should be reserved as alternative therapy.

After a patient—especially an older adult—uses one of these medications for a few months, the patient or caregiver should review the medication with the provider to determine if it can be reduced and eventually stopped, particularly if the acute episode that was the catalyst for the prescription has resolved.

Antipsychotics	
Second Generation	aripiprazole, clozapine, iloperidone, lurasidone, olanzapine, paliperidone, pimavanserin, quetiapine, risperidone, ziprasidone
First Generation	haloperidol

► **ASK: After a few months of use and every few months there after, if the medication is still necessary.**

- Especially if the patient is experiencing falls, dizziness or lightheadedness when getting up from lying down or sitting.
- If the patient has cardiovascular changes—palpitations, slow or fast heart rate, worsening arrhythmias.
- If the medication is providing any benefit.

  NOTE: These medications would need to be tapered slowly when decreasing or stopping.

Antiseizure or Anticonvulsants

Antiseizure medications are used to reduce seizure activity. Some of these medications are also used as mood stabilizers in people with bipolar disorder and for nerve pain, also called neuropathy.

Information on when and how to reduce or deprescribe antiseizure medications is minimal at best. I have personally counseled patients in their 70s who had been taking antiseizure medicines since they had a seizure when they were in their 20s, although they had never experienced another episode. Antiseizure medications are prescribed to reduce the risk of seizure relapse, and a patient who has experienced seizures may be apprehensive about reducing or stopping such medications. This is especially true for those who drive and do not want to have a seizure while driving or be forced to stop driving as a temporary precaution if the medication is changed.

Seizure medications can lead to osteoporosis, fatigue, hair loss, liver toxicity, skin reactions, and hematological changes. Risk versus benefit needs to be evaluated.

Antiseizure	
Hydantoin	phenytoin
Miscellaneous	carbamazepine, lamotrigine, levetiracetam, oxcarbazepine, topiramate, valproic acid, zonisamide

► **ASK: Do I still need to take antiseizure meds?**

- How can I slowly taper off my anti-seizure meds?

Benzodiazepines

Benzodiazepines are medications used to reduce anxiety and enhance sleep. They tend to be used episodically and on an as-needed basis when someone may be suffering from insomnia or feeling anxious.

Benzodiazepines are best to be used only minimally and should be reduced and eventually deprescribed, as they can affect cognition and increase confusion and fall risk. If you suffer from chronic anxiety or have had multiple anxious episodes throughout the years, you should talk to your health-care provider about other types of medication that are more suited to long-term use rather than taking a benzodiazepine for each episode. Think about it: reducing the occurrence of anxiety/panic episodes may in itself make you feel better. Other medications for chronic anxiety include some of the ones highlighted in the antidepressant category, including the SSRIs sertraline and citalopram, for example.

Benzoiazepines
alprazolam, chonazepam, diazepam, lorazepam, oxazepam, temazepam, triazolam

► **ASK: How can I taper off this medicine?**

- I have had anxiety chronically, is there a medicine I can take that will help reduce my anxious feeling so that I am not treating each episode?
- I am concerned about falls, is this a medication that I can stop to reduce my risk?

Bisphosphonates

Bisphosphonates are used to build bone and improve bone density. They are regularly prescribed to offset the effects of osteoporosis or bone cancer.

Sometimes medications are continued beyond the time in which even the medication's own guidelines would say it should be stopped, as is the case with bisphosphonates, which have a timeline of use. The first evaluation to consider, whether these medications should be continued, is at the three-year mark. If your bone density has not increased enough at that point and/or you are still at high risk for a fracture, then the medication may be continued and reevaluated every two years, for up to 10 years, maximum. Beyond 10 years, bisphosphonates are not therapeutically helpful and cause more side effects, such as stomach and esophagus ulcers, difficulty swallowing, heartburn, and muscle and bone pain.

Bisphosphonates
alendronate, ibandronate, risedronate, zolendronic acid

► **ASK: How long should I take this medicine?**

- How long have I been taking this medication?
- When should I have my bone density checked?

Blood Pressure Medications

Blood pressure medications are also called antihypertensives. There are many categories of this type of medication, which are used to reduce blood pressure and typically need to be taken indefinitely for continued blood pressure control.

Blood pressure medications can be beneficial in reducing progression of heart disease, heart attacks, strokes, and the risk of kidney disease. Multiple medications may be necessary to lower blood pressure; however, those medications need to be reduced or removed as people age. Blood pressure goals can also vary and become less stringent with age, health status, and patient sensitivity to side effects.

Some blood pressure medications, such as diuretics, can cause lightheadedness, dizziness, low blood pressure, decreased heart rate, dehydration, or electrolyte imbalance, all of which increase the risk of falls, injury, or other cardiovascular events. Such symptoms may call for a reduction in the medication.

Calcium channel blockers can increase the risk of edema, causing swollen feet and ankles, a condition that is especially concerning in people who have heart failure. Adjusting blood pressure medications by reducing or stopping the calcium channel blocker may reduce the risk of heart failure exacerbation that can lead to hospitalizations.

Blood Pressure Medications	
ACE inhibitors	benazepril, captopril, enalapril, lisinopril, quinapril
ARBs	irbesartan, losartan, olmesartan, valsartan,
Beta-blockers	atenolol, metoprolol, nebivolol
Calcium channel blockers	amlodipine, diltiazem, verapamil
Diuretics:	
Loop	bumetanide, ethacrynic acid, furosemide, torsemide
Potassium-sparing	amiloride, eplerenone, spironolactone, triamterene
Thiazide	chlorthalidone, hydrochlorothiazide

► **ASK: Could a medication I take cause the swollen ankles that I experience?**

- What is an ideal blood pressure goal for me?
- Could my medicine be causing me to feel lightheaded or dizzy even though I have been taking it for years?

Dementia Medications

Dementia medications help to slow the progression of cognitive deficits. There are many forms of dementia, with the most common being Alzheimer's disease.

These medications can be one of the most difficult groups of medications to deprescribe, and it is estimated that a third of dementia medications are unnecessarily continued. Dementia medications are tricky. Not everyone responds to them, and they can trigger several side effects. And the medications often have no therapeutic benefit after a time, even for people who were helped by them initially.

Side effects of dementia meds include urinary incontinence, diarrhea, runny nose, falls, arrhythmias, slowed heart rate. Patients tend to be treated for these issues with other medications.

Dementia Medications	
Acetylcholinesterase inhibitors	donepezil, galantamine, rivastigmine
NMDA receptor antagonist	memantine

► **ASK: How long should I take this medication?**

- How will we determine if the medication is still working?
- Could I be taking other medications due to side effects of these meds?

Diabetes Medications

There are two types of diabetes: type 1 and type 2. Type 1 diabetes means the body is not making insulin; therefore, the only treatment is insulin. Type 2 diabetes is more complex in that insulin is made but not used efficiently by the body; therefore, other medications are needed to support the use of insulin, produce more insulin, or reduce glucose release and availability. Type 2 diabetes can progress to the point of requiring insulin use, but it can also be reversed through lifestyle changes, including reducing weight; balancing nutrition of carbohydrates, fats, and proteins; and increasing activity levels.

When treating either type of diabetes, it is important to be aware of hypoglycemia, or low blood sugar, which can cause you to feel shaky, confused, or moody and increase your heart rate. Sugar is needed immediately to treat a hypoglycemic episode, and you can get it by taking glucose tablets, hard candy, honey, juice, or soda. Hypoglycemia can quickly cause a person to lose consciousness, which can increase falls and require a trip to the emergency department. As they age, people taking medications for diabetes may become more susceptible to hypoglycemic episodes and may have reduced awareness of warning signs. Or patients may need less medication over time if they lose weight or have other changes in their body.

Diabetes Medications	
Biguanide	metformin
DDP-4 inhibitors	linagliptin, saxagliptin, sitagliptin
GLP-1	dulaglutide, exenatide, liraglutide, semaglutide
Insulin	insulin-aspart, -degludec, -detemir, -glargine, -lispro, -NPH, regular
Meglitinide	nateglinide, repaglinide
SGLT2 inhibitor	canagliflozin, dapagliflozin, empagliflozin
Sulfonylureas	glipizide, glyburide, glimepiride
Thiazolidinedione	pioglitazone, rosiglitazone

► **ASK: What is my ideal A1c goal?**

- How can I prevent blood sugar lows?
- What lifestyle measures can I work towards to reduce my need for my type 2 diabetes medications?

Diphenhydramine

Diphenhydramine and other over-the-counter (OTC) antihistamines—especially the first-generation products (the ones that have been around for years)—are used in medicines to alleviate allergies, in sleep aids, and night-time cough and cold medicines.

OTC products, including pain relief medicines, "PM" or other nighttime products, antihistamines, cough and cold products, and sleep aids typically contain an active ingredient called diphenhydramine (pronounced di-fen-hi-dra-mean.) Diphenhydramine can cause a multitude of side effects, especially in older adults, and it lasts many hours longer in their bodies than it does in younger adults. Side effects include dry eyes, dry mouth, and difficulty urinating. It can also cause sleepiness (hence the reason it is used in nighttime products), but this sleepiness can last longer in older adults, resulting in an effect that many people describe as a "hangover" the morning after taking a diphenhydramine product. Other side effects include slowed cognition, confusion, and increased heart rate, which can trigger possible arrhythmias and increase the risk of falls.

When I see diphenhydramine on a patient's list of medications, I always question the need. This is one medication that older adults should avoid.

Antihistamines	
First Generation	brompheniramine, chlorpheniramine, clemastine, diphenhydramine, doxylamine, meclizine
Second Generation	cetirizine, fexofenadine, loratadine

► **THINK about Good Sleep Hygiene:**

- Less caffeine, especially later in the day- that includes chocolate too!
- More exercise during the day.
- Have your last meal / snack 2 hours before bedtime.
- De-stimulate through the evening hours, less screen-time.

► **ASK: If a medication you take could be keeping you awake.**

- Are you taking your medications at the right time so it does not interfere with sleep?

____

____

____

____

____

Eye Drops for Glaucoma

When using eye drops, use only one drop at a time, close eye tight or place your finger in the corner of your eye by the bridge of your nose to block your tear duct for one minute. This allows the eye drop to work within your eye.

Few people realize that eye drops can have effects on their whole body. When using eye drops, use only one drop at a time, close eye tight or place your finger in the corner of your eye by the bridge of your nose to block your tear duct for one minute. This allows the eye drop to work within your eye.

Timolol, an eye drop to fight glaucoma, should be used in this manner to reduce possible systemic effects. Timolol is a nonselective beta-blocker that may slow the heart rate or constrict the airways of the lungs. These effects can cause dizziness, chest discomfort, shortness of breath, and—you guessed it—falls.

Dorzolamide, another eye drop used for glaucoma, needs to be eliminated from your system, as all medications do. It is not recommended for use in patients with severe kidney dysfunction, as it can cause increased side effects including anemia and other blood, liver, and skin disorders.

Eye drops for Glaucoma	
Carbonic anhydrase inhibitors	brinzolamide, dorzolamide
Beta blocker	timolol
Prostaglandin analog	bimatoprost, latanoprost, travoprost

- **ASK: If your kidney function is within the parameters to use the carbonic anhydrase inhibitor eye drops, brinzolamide or dorzolamide.**
  - Ask if slowed heart rate or shortness of breath could be from the timolol eye drops.

Gabapentin/GABA Analog

Gabapentin, originally approved for seizures, is typically used for neuropathic pain, including diabetic neuropathy, and nerve pain from shingles.

Some medications may need a change in dosing as well as frequency, depending upon a user's age, kidney function, and/or liver function. Gabapentin is one medication that needs to be dosed carefully, especially in older adults, as kidney function can negatively affect its elimination, increasing the risk of falls and side effects.

Gabapentin has quite a range of dosing, especially for nerve pain (neuropathy). Maximum daily doses for generally healthy adults with good working kidneys is 3,600 mg per 24 hours. Typically, this is taken in divided doses of 1,200 mg three times throughout the day. For someone on hemodialysis (a process that filters an individual's blood if one's kidneys are unhealthy and unable to do so), the dose drops to 300 mg three times per week. That's quite a significant difference in dosing!

GABA analog
Gabapentin, pregabalin

► **ASK: Is the gabapentin dosed appropriately for my kidney function?**

- Is gabapentin causing fluid /swelling in your ankles?
- Is gabapentin truly helping or are you taking it because no one has asked if you still have pain or if it helps relieve your pain?

Nonsteroidal Anti-Inflammatory Drugs (NSAIDs)

NSAIDs can be found in OTC or prescription products that help alleviate pain, inflammation, and fever. NSAIDs are available in prescription strength, prescription medication combinations, and widely available in both single and combination OTC products.

People reach for OTC pain relief for sore muscles, back pain, headaches, knee pain, or general aches. These can be obtained at the grocery store, gas station, or pharmacy, and from family and friends. NSAIDs, including ibuprofen, naproxen, and aspirin, for example, are marketed under various brand names and are included in combination medications such as pain relief for migraines, cough and cold, and allergy medications.

And because many of these are sold without prescriptions, we think they are safe for anyone to take. This is far from true, and many people wind up in the hospital every year because of problems caused or worsened by NSAIDs. People with kidney disease, heart failure, or hypertension especially need to be aware that NSAIDs can make their conditions worse.

NSAIDs
diclofenac, ibuprofen, naproxen, meloxicam

► **ASK: Is it okay to take NSAIDs? – Especially if you have stomach problems, heart issues, kidney problems, or diabetes.**

- Does the medication you are taking for headaches, cough, cold, and other OTCs have an NSAID included in their active agents?
- If you should stop taking NSAIDs before a procedure.

Proton Pump Inhibitors (PPIs)

Proton pump inhibitors reduce the acid in the stomach to help alleviate acid reflux, heartburn, and ulcers. Over the past few decades, long-term use of PPIs has become a far too common way to treat gastroesophageal reflux disease (GERD), also known as gastric reflux or acid reflux. PPIs should be used only for a short period of time, approximately two weeks, to resolve this acute condition. Many people, however, have remained on these medications for years.

There are many uses for PPIs including prophylactically in the hospital to prevent ulcers or to prevent a stomach or gastrointestinal (GI) bleed for people on blood thinners. PPIs may also be prescribed for more significant gastric acid conditions such as Barrett's esophagus. However, if chronic conditions do not exist, then the PPI is not needed indefinitely.

Why is it important to stop a PPI if it is not needed? PPIs increase the pH of the stomach, making it less acidic. This increased pH interrupts the absorption of many nutrients that need a more acidic environment. These nutrients include vitamin B12, vitamin D, magnesium, calcium, and iron, and all play an important role in your general well-being.

Proton Pump Inhibitors (PPIs)
dexlansoprazole, esomeprazole, lansoprazole, omeprazole, pantoprazole, rabeprazole

► **ASK: What are my magnesium, iron, vitamin D, and B12 levels? Especially if you have been taking a PPI for a year or more.**

- How do I taper off a PPI so that I do not experience acid rebound?
- What changes can I make to reduce acid reflux?—Such as:
    - Foods to avoid or to eat
    - Timing of eating and then lying down
    - Amount of food / portion control
    - Exercise

____

____

____

____

____

Statins

Statins reduce total cholesterol, increase HDL (the "good" cholesterol), and decrease LDL (the "bad" cholesterol). Keeping cholesterol in check helps cardiovascular (heart) health.

The idea of deprescribing statins has become a controversial topic. Some studies show stopping statins may cause an increased risk of hospitalization and poor cardiovascular outcomes over time.[17, 18] Reviewing other studies with shorter time results, stopping the statin for 60 days, showed to be acceptable, while stopping a statin for two years time showed to be more problematic.[19] Older adults may benefit from continuing statins because cardiovascular risks increase with age; however, many studies on this issue do not have data for people older than 75 years to show whether the benefits outweigh the risks. Deprescribing statins should be individualized, with patient and provider considering adverse side effects, drug interactions, and life expectancy while determining the appropriateness of continuing the medication.

Statins have been shown to potentially cause muscle weakness over time in aging adults.[20] The weakness may occur so gradually that users may not realize that a medication could be causing the problem. But any medication that may contribute to muscle weakness could lead to reduced exercise and eventually falls. If someone is experiencing such problems, it could be time to consider reducing the statin to a lower dose and reevaluating cholesterol levels, muscle strength, and pain/discomfort.

Statins
atorvastatin, fluvastatin, lovastatin, pitavastatin, pravastatin, rosuvastatin, simvastatin

► **ASK: What are my ideal cholesterol goals?**

- Could a lower dose of statin make me less achy and still be effective?
- Could fish oil be preventing me from getting to my LDL goal?

Tramadol

Tramadol is used for acute or chronic pain management. It is part of the opioid family and used for moderate to moderately severe pain.Tramadol is being discussed here because it is often believed to be a better option to treat pain in older adults. However, that is not always true.

I was asked to review the medications of an older male by his daughter, who said her father was just not "bouncing back" to his normal self after a recent surgery. She stated he was typically a very bright man—he had worked as a scientist for many years—who did not have dementia. When I reviewed his medications, I noticed that tramadol was being prescribed four weeks post-surgery. He had not been on this medication previously. In discussing this medication with the daughter, I learned she was not quite certain if the medication was helping with pain or if her dad even had pain any longer. We decided she would work with the doctor to taper the tramadol and eventually deprescribe the med. When we spoke a couple of weeks later, she told me her father was off the tramadol, back to his bright self, and not experiencing pain, and she thanked me for helping her and her father.

Opioids
oxycodone, hydrocodone, morphine, tramadol

► **ASK: Is this medication appropriate and for how long?**

- How do I decide if I need to take it or not?
- What other medications should not be taken with these medications?

Other Surprises You Might Find in Your Pillbox

A careful examination of your pill box may turn up drugs that interact badly with each other or prescriptions that exceed the maximum dosing for your age. Here are some examples of problems you might find.

Drug-drug interactions

- ► **ASK: To have a medication review, find a pharmacist to review.**
  - Use steps 1-5 of the Medication Optimization Plan (MOP)

Drug-disease interactions

- ► **ASK: If any of the medications you take might be worsening another condition you have.**

Maximum dosing problems

- ► **ASK: If you are taking the correct dose for all of your meds—even those you have taken for years.**

Medications that need special attention

- Diabetes medications
- Levothyroxine
- Digoxin
- Warfarin

► **THINK about a monitoring schedule; have labs checked if the manufacturer changes**

Hazardous medication combinations

- Benzodiazepines, muscle relaxants, and opioids
- Benzodiazepines and opioids
- Gabapentin and opioids
- Multiple medications that affect the central nervous system

► **CHECK your medication list for these combinations**

What medications in your pill box do you find surprising?

____

____

____

____

____

____

____

____

What are your concerns?

____

____

____

____

____

____

____

____

____

____

____

Falls, Frailty, and Transitions of Care

Falls

IN REAL LIFE

Falls and Deprescribing

Mrs. D has a history of falls, including multiple times in one day. Her medication list follows: acetaminophen PM (for pain and sleep aid), atenolol (for heart rate and blood pressure), duloxetine (for depression and nerve pain), fentanyl (for pain), gabapentin (for neuropathy), glimepiride (for diabetes), lisinopril (for blood pressure), lovastatin (for cholesterol), mirtazapine (an antipsychotic / antidepressant), ropinirole (for restless leg), and trazodone (for insomnia and depression). Eight of these 11 medications can increase the risk of falls: acetaminophen PM, duloxetine, fentanyl, gabapentin, glimepiride, mirtazapine, ropinirole, and trazodone.

The remaining medications are not listed as high-fall-risk, but atenolol and lisinopril could contribute to a potential fall due to cardiovascular side effects, and lovastatin could contribute to a potential fall due to possible muscle weakness. In addition, many of these medications can cause cognitive deficits, which can cause a patient to become easily confused and take incorrect medications or incorrect dosages, possibly doubling up on medications by accident. You can see the culmination of possibilities that may cause harm for this patient and may be contributing to her many falls.

As has been pointed out throughout this workbook, the effects of medications can be additive, so a person's risk of falling increases when taking multiple medications that increase their risk of falls. Therefore, it's not necessarily one medication, but two or more medications together that could drive up fall risk. Using lowest possible doses and deprescribing unnecessary and duplicate medications can help lower the risk of falls.

The following table shows the precautions of Mrs. D's medication list based on various criteria. Perhaps deprescribing some medication by stopping and reducing others may be beneficial to reduce Mrs. D's falls. A health-care provider could first target acetaminophen PM, mirtazapine, or fentanyl, as these meds are each potentially inappropriate according to all three criteria reviewed.

Mrs. D's Medications and Potential for Inappropriateness

Medication	Beers	STOPP	STEADI
Acetaminophen PM	x	x	x
Atenolol		x	x
Duloxetine	x		x
Fentanyl	x	x	x
Gabapentin	x		x
Glimepiride	x		
Lisinopril			x
Lovastatin			
Mirtazapine	x	x	x
Ropinirole			x
Trazodone			x

Beers[21], STOPP [22], and STEADI[23] are reliable resources that highlight medications that need to be avoided or used with caution, especially in older adults, due to potential increased risk of falls. More can be learned about these in the Resources Guide at the end of the book.

Frailty

There are several tools available to measure frailty. Frailty ranges from "Fit to Frail". Some scores or index range from 0-3; 0-5; 1-5; 1-7; or 1-9. No matter the scale or the numbers you use to determine frailty know:

- **The higher the number on the index means increased frailty.**
- **The number can vary—that is improve or worsen.**
- **Dementia increases frailty scores.**

MedStrong Frailty Scale

< 1 2 3 4 5 6 7 8 9 10 >

Very Fit > Somewhat fit > Somewhat Frail > Concerningly Frail > Frail

Very fit means no assistive devices, able to do everything for themselves, exercises regularly, and most likely is helping others.

Somewhat fit is able to be independent, no assistive devices, able to move well.

Somewhat frail may need an assistive device, may need some light assistance with daily activities, cleaning/household chores.

Concerningly frail needs assistance with many household chores and daily activities such as dressing, bathing, food preparation, has a history of falls.

Frail is unable to be independent at all, bedridden, 24/7 round the clock care for all needs.

How does someone improve frailty?

By reducing unnecessary and inappropriate medications; exercise that can even start with lying in bed exercises, seated exercises, and increasing ability as strength improves; nutritional intake including protein, fats, and carbohydrates.

What is my frailty score? ___________

How can I reduce the the risk of worsening frailty?

____

____

____

Transitions of Care

One key component of successful transitions of care is reducing readmissions back to the hospital, especially within 30 days of being discharged no matter if for the same reason or something else. Below is a process as to how to reduce readmissions.[24]

Reducing Readmissions

- ***Reconcile the medication list.***
  That is be certain you understand what meds you need to take, what you need to stop, and to be certain if you are unclear on any medication that you have at home that you check first if it is still needed.
- ***Employ patient-centered education by the pharmacist during the hospital stay.***
  In some hospitals pharmacists visit with patients to review medications, if this is available take the time to ask questions and write notes.
- ***Ensure the patient has access to needed medications at discharge.***
  If you are starting a new medication after a hospitalization, be certain that it is covered by your insurance, that you can afford it, and that you are able to pick it up from the pharmacy or have it delivered.
- ***Counsel the patient post-discharge.***
  After discharge from the hospital, you may receive a call from the hospital or the care group that will follow you, ask questions if needed. Have your questions ready!
- ***The patient remains home and avoids readmission.***
  That is the hope that your transition is successful, and you are able to reduce the risk of falls and improve your frailty score.

What medications have you been uncertain of during transitions of care?

____

____

____

What medications have you started due to a hospitalization that you wonder if it is still necessary?

____

____

____

What medications in your pill box might contribute to falls or frailty or were changed due to transitions in care?

____

____

____

____

What are your concerns?

____

____

____

____

____

Educated, Enlightened, Empowered

Wait....What? Just like any other change or non-change, medications need to be constantly reviewed. Remember that Step 5 of the ***MedStrong Medication Optimization Plan (MOP)*** requires monitoring, documentation, and follow-up. Embrace that deprescribing is a constant consideration just like health checks, lifestyle changes, and taking helpful medications appropriately. If you "DO," you will be empowered to take a more active role in maintaining your health.

This section has touched on a plethora of information and thrown around a lot of tongue-twister names that may not be familiar to anyone who is not working in the health-care industry. But it hopefully has enlightened you and illustrated to patients and health-care providers alike that many familiar medications can cause problems and that the risk-benefit analysis differs from person to person.

Use what you have learned here and keep reviewing your medications with all your health-care providers to optimize your medications and your health outcomes. Remember that deprescribing can be a beneficial treatment option that can make you feel and function better and may even alleviate a geriatric syndrome that concerns you or, better yet, avoid one altogether!

In Part III we will explore more potential concerns that can occur and also see that not all changes are necessarily correct and appropriate.

Overview of Part II: What Can We DO? Deprescribe to Optimize!

- Deprescribe to optimize (DO) is a thoughtful process that is shared between patients, caregivers, and health-care providers, including pharmacists, the medication experts.
- DO involves multiple conversations, action steps, monitoring, and documenting throughout the continuum of care.
- Prescribing and deprescribing use the same thought process: adding or subtracting a medication is an individualized, step-by-step process that requires monitoring to judge outcomes.
- The ***MedStrong Medication Optimization Plan (MOP)*** and the multiple MedStrong checklists provided in this book can help patients and providers successfully complete the deprescribing process. Extra forms are available at the end of this workbook.
- Listing the medications you take and considering if each medication is effective, necessary, or added due to side effects is an important first step of MOP.
- Knowing the right questions to ask at the right time and in the right situation will help empower individuals to optimize their medications.
- Consider with your health-care providers if stopping, changing, or reducing a medication is a good therapeutic plan.
- Plan and be ready to monitor, document, and follow up on the steps in your plan.
- Know what's in your pill box. Being educated so that you can become your own best advocate is key to taking control of your health outcomes.
- As your body changes, consider the potential for side effects of various medications and the hazards of particular combinations.
- Deprescribing and optimizing medications can reduce hospitalizations, falls, and other adverse effects.

Many medications that are beneficial—even life-saving— for some people can be harmful to others. Prescribing and deprescribing should be part of a thoughtful, informed process with patients, caregivers, and health-care providers making decisions based on an individual's unique life circumstances. DO takes effort, but DO-ing keeps us enlightened, energized, accountable, and learning for the good of ourselves and others.

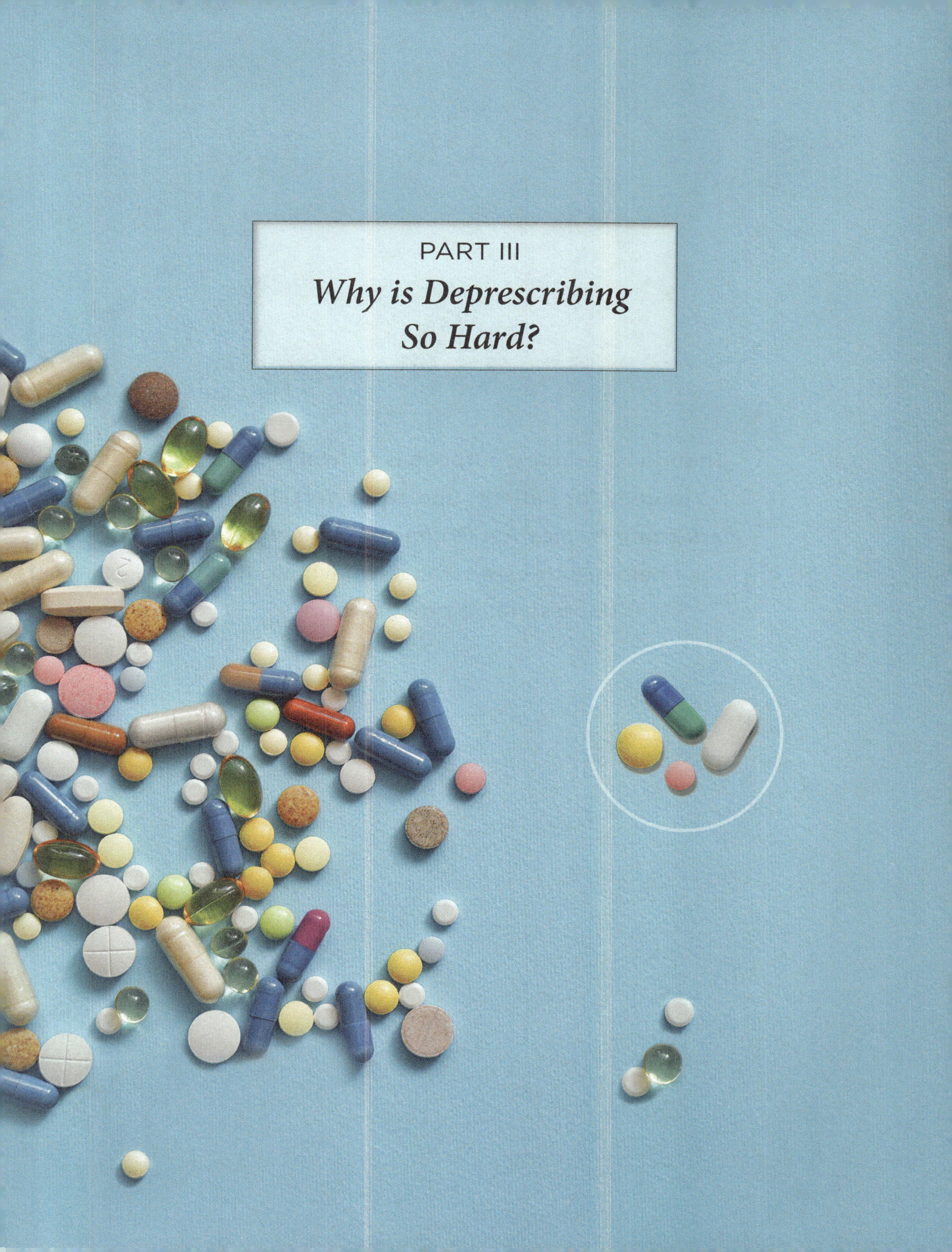

PART III
Why is Deprescribing So Hard?

“

Though its primary purpose is to facilitate the journey for patients and caregivers, the ***MedStrong Medication Optimization Plan (MOP)*** can help health-care providers navigate the deprescribing process too.

Deprescribing in a Prescribing World

THIS SECTION PROVIDES A PERSPECTIVE of deprescribing from the prescribers' point of view and barriers that affect both patients and providers.

Each patient case is individualized and requires monitoring and evaluation if a medication is necessary or if it can be deprescribed. When reviewing medications, I use the Medication Appropriateness Index[25, 26] as a guide to assessing each medication. This list of 10 questions serves as a map to make sense of medications being taken and to formulate questions to determine if a medication is indeed appropriate. These questions help determine if any adjustments may be necessary.

Medication Appropriateness Index	
Indication	What is the medication being used for?
Effect	Is the medication effective for this use?
Dose	Is this dose correct?
Instructions	Are the directions correct?
Drug-drug Interactions	Are there drug-drug interactions of concern?
Drug-disease Interactions	Can the medication make another condition worse?
Duplications	Is the medication similar to another?
Practical	Can the patient use/take the medication properly?
Duration	How long should/how long has the drug been being taken?
Affordable	Is this the least expensive medication the patient could be taking for their condition?

Potentially Inappropriate Meds for Older Adults

Potential Innapropriate Category	Example
Original indication (health concern) no longer applies	During a hospitalization, the patient was given a medication, such as a proton pump inhibitor (e.g., omeprazole), to prevent gastric acid and ulcers while hospitalized. The patient is still taking the medication a year later, without an indication or need for the med.
Drug-drug interactions	A patient is taking amlodipine for blood pressure and simvastatin 40mg for cholesterol. Since amlodipine can increase the drug availability of simvastatin, it is recommended that the simvastatin be reduced to 20mg to reduce the drug-drug interaction and potential muscle ache and pain side effects the patient may encounter or already experience.
Drug-disease interactions	A patient experiences knee pain from walking and decides to take ibuprofen. The patient has heart failure and begins to retain fluids, experiences swollen ankles, and becomes short of breath. The ibuprofen has caused an exacerbation of heart failure. Providers should advise patients to avoid ibuprofen and similar products for future episodes of pain and make recommendations about what can be taken.
Inappropriate treatment for patient life expectancy	An 85-year-old patient with type 2 diabetes is experiencing many episodes of low blood sugar (hypoglycemia). His A1c is 7%. The provider decides to stop one of the medications used to treat diabetes and tells the patient, A1c could go as high as 8.5% without concern. Although lower A1c levels are important in younger patients to protect smaller blood vessels, the higher A1c is less risky than hypoglycemic (low blood sugar) episodes in older patients.
Medication no longer aligns with goals	A patient would prefer to be on less medication, experience fewer side effects, and have a better daily quality of life than be on higher doses at therapeutic goals, which could extend life but leave them unable to enjoy their favorite activities.
Medication poses high risk of falls/ traffic accidents	Zolpidem, used for sleep, can cause falls, traffic accidents, and confusion, especially in older patients. Advise a patient to reduce caffeine and chocolate, exercise regularly, and avoid electronics at bedtime to improve sleep and eliminate need for zolpidem at bedtime.
Experiencing an adverse effect	A patient being treated for pain with tramadol has a seizure. Tramadol should be stopped, as it can lower seizure threshold. Better to deprescribe a medication than to add medications for a side effect.

A Closer Look: Insomnia Medications

An article highlighting an interview with Dr. Kevin Pottie, associate professor of the Departments of Family Medicine and Epidemiology & Community Medicine at the University of Ottawa, offers glimpses of the problems of polypharmacy for insomnia treatment.[27] Insomnia medications can cause cognitive impairment, falls, and traffic accidents. Not only that, their effectiveness over a long period of time is questionable.

There are also confusing dosing restrictions of some medications for insomnia, such as zolpidem. Zolpidem should be dosed at 5 mg at bedtime for women and all older adults regardless of gender, and dosed at 10 mg at bedtime for younger adult males. The use of these medications in older adults is cautioned against in many of the criteria available including the Beers Criteria, STOPP and START, CDC-STEADI, and Choosing Wisely.

If someone really cannot sleep, what should be done for them? More and more studies are showing the benefits of nonmedication approaches, such as encouraging better sleep hygiene and counseling, including cognitive behavior therapy. Improving sleep hygiene may include reducing foods and activities that may cause insomnia, such as caffeine and chocolate, and avoiding napping during the day and screen time later in the day or evening.

Dr. Pottie mentions that instead of getting caught in the cycle of finding a medication to treat a patient's insomnia, health-care providers should first review current medications that may be causing the insomnia. It could be the timing of medications or some other underlying issue such as pain, sleep apnea, or anxiety that could be keeping the patient awake.

The Targeted Approach

Another approach to deprescribing is to begin by targeting one group of health issues. For example, begin with medications that have significant side effects, such as anticholinergics, increased risk of falls, or cognition effects. Next, target legacy prescriptions: medications that should be prescribed only for a moderate length of time, not indefinitely. Or review specific medications first, such as antiseizure meds, proton pump inhibitors (PPIs), or gabapentin. This approach can be especially beneficial when a provider is hindered by time constraints. The categories illustrated in the previous table can be good areas to target in this approach.

Pause and Monitor

Pause and monitor is another approach to deprescribing, and it calls for patients and prescribers to work together to decide if a medication is actually necessary, especially if there is question of risk versus benefit. Pause and monitor allows both parties to commit to the idea of deprescribing, while also committing to follow up to determine the results.[28] This process can be especially helpful when either the patient or the provider is leery about stopping a medication. Including a "pause and monitor" clause in any deprescribing approach may make it easier for the patient and provider to share in the decision-making process.

Another way providers can help make the deprescribing process easier is by asking patients questions that ensure they are involved in the process. These questions include

What matters to you?

____

____

____

____

Is deprescribing something you would consider?

____

____

____

What medications are important to you and why?

____

____

____

What options would you like to have?

____

____

____

____

Team Approach

All of these approaches demonstrate that deprescribing should be an individualized, multilayer process that involves cooperation between the patient, providers, and caregivers. This cooperation plays a key role in whether the deprescribing process succeeds.

Think about it: if a patient, caregiver, or pharmacist approaches a doctor about deprescribing and the doctor dismisses the request without a good explanation, then they are not working as a team. If a doctor makes an effort to inform the pharmacy that a medication was deprescribed, but the pharmacy does not update the patient's records and continues to make medication refills available, then the team approach has been dismissed. Because there are so many scenarios that can stop deprescribing in its tracks, it sometimes requires multiple attempts to succeed.

The deprescribing process should be a pragmatic, methodical, and monitored team effort, and if one member or part of the team effort breaks down, the whole process can also break down. Primary care providers, specialists, and pharmacists all need to be on board, willing to communicate, and able to make changes effectively. Without a team effort, one provider may recommend a change that does not get carried forth.

For example, automatic prescription refills can derail a deprescribing effort. A provider tells a patient to stop taking a medication, but a refill of the medication becomes available at the pharmacy a few weeks later. The patient may become confused and think the doctor ordered the medication again. Health-care providers need to be able to communicate changes to multiple team members to ensure the changes are made in all arms of the system, rather than expecting the patient to make the system work.

What medications do you have on auto-refill—are they all still necessary?

Auto-refilled Medications

Medication	Continue	Call Pharmacy to Stop

Changing the Culture

The growing evidence for the benefits of deprescribing in health outcomes, quality of life, and cost containment calls for a cultural change that will expect deprescribing to be integrated into the process the moment a medication is prescribed. "Life-long medications" should be a thing of the past.[29] Instead, providers should establish a time span to review medications and either continue therapy or stop therapy as part of the health-care protocol. Adding a commitment to deprescribing should be considered in every patient encounter.

Deprescribing does not mean health-care providers give up on their patients, stop all their medications, and stop prescribing for preventive purposes. Instead, deprescribing is another way of managing risks and benefits while considering many factors that influence good medicine. It takes skill to look at a patient's health changes and realize the moment when a medicine is no longer efficacious or when it begins to pose an unacceptable risk or burden.

Currently, there is minimal professional guidance to help health-care providers know when to stop medications or how to determine whether harm may occur over time if medications are or are not stopped. Studies are necessary to evaluate these outcomes, but who should be responsible for studying these factors? Will a manufacturer be on board with studying the best ways to stop medications? Should we have both prescribing information and deprescribing information for all medications?

What about the patient goals within these guidelines? When is it time to stop a medication for a patient? Do we wait for the hospitalization, the fall, the adverse event before we intervene? Perhaps there needs to be a deprescribing treatment plan within the treatment guidelines, but further study is needed before that can be done.

Health-care providers do not want to remove medications that are providing benefit and certainly do not want to swing the pendulum from overtreatment to undertreatment. Taking small steps, reevaluating, and monitoring the patient throughout the deprescribing process does take time, but it allows for intervention if necessary.

Providers should also recognize that in the process of deprescribing, "no change" in how the patient is doing can be a good outcome, which is an odd idea for medical professionals accustomed to trying to effect a change. But a patient who stops taking a medication and experiences no change in a condition may very well be counted as a successful deprescribing outcome.

Many medications are intended for chronic, indefinite use; however, labeling a medication as a "lifetime" medication can be inappropriate. As suggested in the "Reducing Inappropriate Polypharmacy" article, medications should be labeled "best before" and then reevaluated for continuation after that date.[30] When counseling patients, health-care providers can tell them that certain medications may need to be taken indefinitely but also warn them that there may very well be a time when discontinuation is warranted.

Providers and patients alike can use the ***MedStrong Annual Physical Med Checklist*** (see the form on the next page) to make this process easier. Each line includes a check box to "Deprescribe" or "Continue," to help foster the idea of thoughtfully reviewing all medications and considering whether it's time to deprescribe.

Barriers to Deprescribing

Patient Barriers:

Check the items you perceive as your barriers to deprescribing.

- ☐ Supplying an accurate, updated list of medications
- ☐ Overwhelmed-uncertain where to begin
- ☐ Uncertainty- (I was told to take this for the rest of my life!)
- ☐ Perception of continued need for medication
- ☐ Unwillingness to ask- (Provider will be upset if asked.)
- ☐ Other ______________________________

Provider Barriers:

Check the items you perceive as your prescriber's barriers to deprescribing.

- ☐ Uncertainty
- ☐ Benefits versus harm
- ☐ Difficult process
- ☐ Lack of evidence / guidelines to deprescribe
- ☐ Not original prescriber
- ☐ Time consuming
- ☐ Other ______________________________

How to Tackle Perceived Barriers:

- ▶ **START SLOWLY:** Pick one med to start with.
- ▶ **ASK:** Each time you are at your appointments.
- ▶ **MAKE:** It part of the health visit.
- ▶ **DISCUSS:** With every provider in every setting.
- ▶ **EDUCATE:** Teach others to have these conversations.
- ▶ **TELL:** Others about ***MedStrong.***

MedStrong Annual Physical Med Checklist

My Medication and Strength	How Taken & When	Reason for the Medication	ACTION - Check the Box That Applies	
			Deprescribe	Continue

Pharma Fails

THROUGHOUT MUCH OF THIS BOOK, we have reviewed the roles that patients, caregivers, pharmacists, and providers play in polypharmacy and the deprescribing process; but individuals are only part of the health-care picture. The pharmaceutical industry, including pharmacy chains and pharmaceutical manufacturers; and the insurance sector, including private, state, and government-run insurances, play large roles in the way medication is prescribed and dispensed in the United States. Just like the patients, caregivers, and prescribers, they also bear some of the polypharmacy burden and should share in the responsibility of making deprescribing easier and safer. In this chapter, we will examine some of the barriers that can make polypharmacy and the deprescribing process more difficult than it should be.

Brand Extensions

Brand extensions are various products with the same brand name. However, the original active agents may not be in some of the brand extension products. Confused? You should be! Below is a chart of some brand extensions. Be certain to provide the full name of the products you take so that the active ingredients are correctly noted.

Brand	Brand /Brand Extension	Active Ingredient
Zantac	Zantac	ranitidine
	Zantac 360	famotidine
Excedrin	Excedrin	acetaminophen
	Excedrin Migraine	acetiminopen, aspirin, caffeine
Claritin	Claritin	loratadine
	Claritin Eye	ketotifen
Advil	Advil	ibuprofen
	Advil Dual Action	ibuprofen and acetaminophen
Visine	Visine Original	Tetrahydrolozine
	Visine Red Eye	Polyethylene Glycol 400, Tetrahydrolozine, Zinc Sulfate
	Visine Allergy Eye	Naphazoline, Pheniramine

What brand extension medications are you taking? What is the active ingredient?

Medication Reviews:

Medication reviews are different than "med-recs" (medication reconciliations). All we need to do is change the "c" in rec to a "v" can we have "med-revs". Medication reviews are a more thorough process than "med-recs" which are matching that the med list matches what the patient actually takes.

Many folks think that their doctors review their medications, when the medical assistant has done a med rec as part of updating the records and checking vitals.

Medication reviews take time, ask your doctor's office for a specific appointment for a med review, or ask your pharmacist if they can take the time to review your medications and get back to you with any issues / concerns.

Medication Therapy Management (MTM):

Medication Therapy Management is a service by Medicare Plans. Not all Medicare recipients are eligible though. Medicare plans decide on eligibility by determining the number of disease states, number of meds, and cost of medications in order to be eligible.

Check with your plan to see if you qualify. But also know that Board Certified Geriatric Pharmacists are available for a fee to provide this service without specific requirements. Check out helpwithmymeds.com to find a BCGP in your area!

Insurance and Prescribing Limitations:

Insurance companies work to contain health care costs. Restricted drug formularies is one type of cost containment. Drug formularies with tiers, prior authorization, quantity limits, and step therapy are applied to help contain costs.

Fragmented Electronic Med Records:

Electronic records are common in the pharmacy, the physician's office, and the hospital. However, these systems are not necessarily integrated and, in fact, are usually not integrated, at least in the United States. That means doctors and pharmacists may be looking at different medication records, but the patients do not realize the discrepancy. For example, a doctor tells a patient to reduce a medication from two tablets daily to one tablet and changes the in-office records. But the doctor does not send in a new prescription to the pharmacy because it is not a new medicine. When the patient gets a refill, it comes with the old instructions for two tablets daily because the pharmacist's records do not integrate with the doctor's records.

Another area of concern occurs during transitions of care. One hospitalist may make a change to a patient's medications during a hospitalization, but at discharge a different hospitalist may continue medications that the patient was taking prior to the hospitalization. Furthermore, if patients are returning to long-term care, medications may be inadvertently continued if they are not officially discontinued.

There are many more scenarios and barriers that could be discussed in this chapter; however, I think it should be clear that many entities play a part in the culture of polypharmacy. This is not all bad news! Medications have helped us live longer and healthier. The good news is that the medication culture has gotten us to this critical point; the bad news is that there is a critical point. In Part IV, we will look at how we move forward, take action, and avoid overmedication, polypharmacy, and geriatric syndromes related to these issues.

How would you benefit from a medication review?

Do you qualify for an MTM? (Check with your drug insurance plan.)

Overview of Part III: Why Is Deprescribing So Hard?

- Though it looks as if it should be easy, deprescribing is filled with barriers constructed by the patient, caregivers, health-care providers, and the health-care system.
- More and more health-care researchers and organizations are warning about the harms of polypharmacy and recommending methods and guidelines to help health-care providers undertake a deprescribing process.
- Many levels of teamwork are needed to successfully implement and execute deprescribing.
- Conversations about deprescribing are best if continued throughout the continuum of care.
- Minimal guidelines are available to determine when a medication may become inappropriate for a patient.
- A patient's health goals are an important factor in shared decision-making to deprescribe.
- When reviewing outcomes of deprescribing, "no change" may be considered a success.
- Brand-name extensions, auto-refills, and insurance industry guidelines can add to the hazards of polypharmacy and make deprescribing more difficult.
- Medication reviews and Medication Therapy Management (MTM) can have great results but are sometimes limited based on health conditions, number and cost of medications, as well as coverage for such services.

Although modern medicine plays a large role in helping us live longer and better, polypharmacy is harming too many people. There are encouraging signs that our modern health-care system is beginning to see the benefits of cultivating a culture of deprescribing in order to take full advantage of our helpful medical advances.

PART IV
The Way Forward

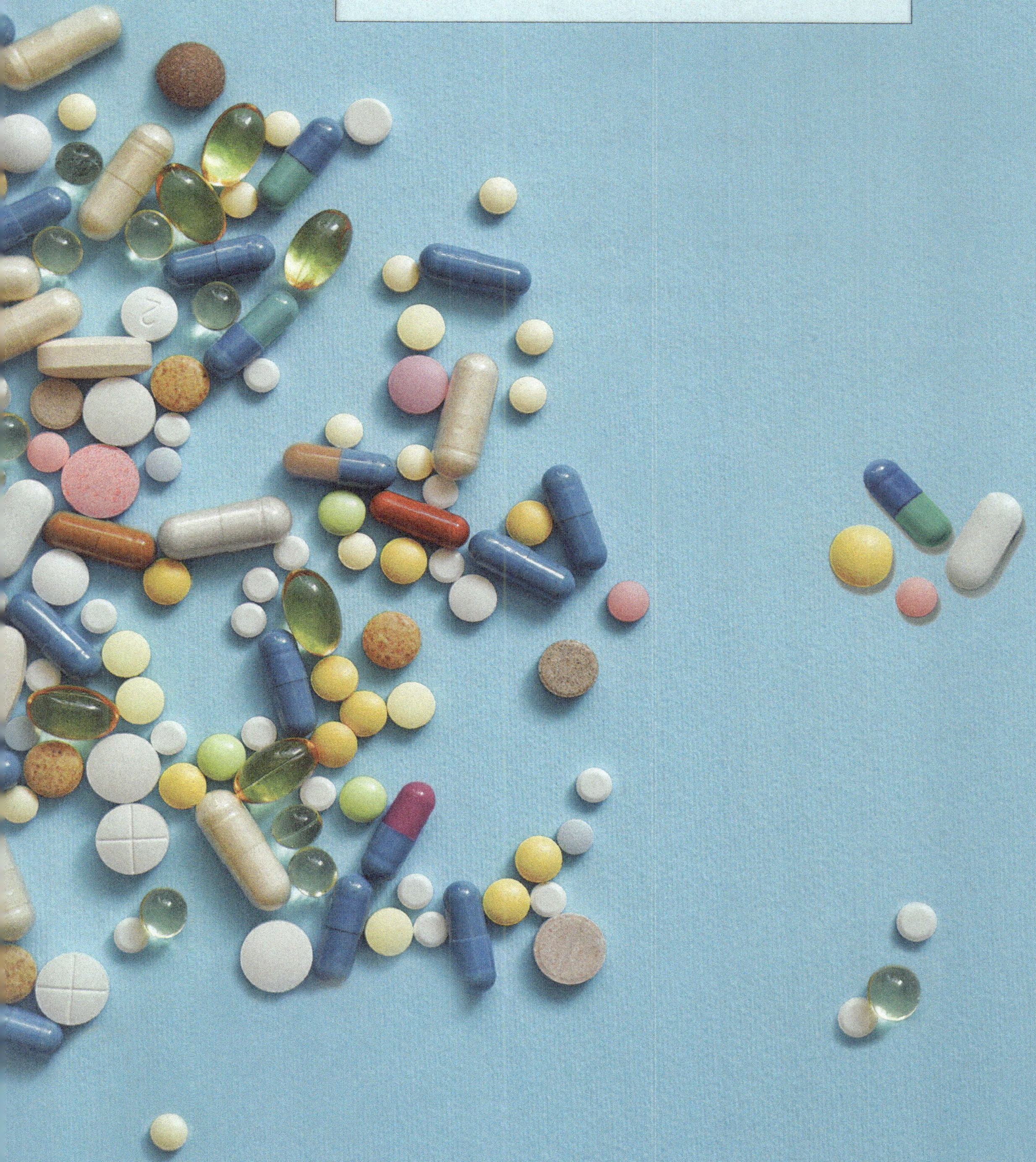

Reviewing medications for need, safety, outcomes, and possible side effects should become routine practice. Now is the time to take action!

Avoiding a MEDisaster

IN THE LATE 1800s SIR WILLIAM OSLER STATED, "The first duty of the physician is to educate the masses not to take medicine."[31] In his 2018 article "What Needs to Change to Make Deprescribing Doable," Dr. Ranit Mishori advocates for deprescribing to be taught along with prescribing in medical school.[32] All of us—patients, caregivers, health-care providers, pharmacists, insurers, and anyone who plays a role in the health system—currently play a part in polypharmacy. Now it's time for all of us to play a part in the deprescribing process.

MedStrong Medication Optimization Plan (MOP)

STEP 1 — **List all Medications.**
Fill out the MedStrong Medication List.

STEP 2 — **Review Medication List.**
Use the MedStrong Medication List and the MedStrong Question List to formulate questions.

STEP 3 — **Decide to Deprescribe with Your Provider.**
Start the "DO" conversation using the Medstrong Question List.

STEP 4 — **Make a Plan.**
Fill out the MedStrong Deprescribing Form.

STEP 5 — **Monitor, Document, Follow-up.**
Use the Medstrong Deprescribing Form and the MedStrong Medication Change Form.

▸ ASK, ASK, ASK

If a medication is switched:

- Double check that the new medication is appropriate
- Be certain to not take the med that is being stopped
- Make certain meds you continue or stop is clear especially during transitions of care
- Update your health records
- Work with your health care professionals—don't forget Step 5

As the Pendulum Swings

Humans are prone to "go all in," and "take it to the max." We encourage each other to "go big or go home." Patience may be a virtue, but we never hear sports fans yelling, "Patience! Patience!" as they cheer on their teams. We like to see immediate results and exceed all of our desired goals. Only in golf do you strive to be subpar! But we should not approach deprescribing with an all-or-nothing mind-set. We do not want to swing the pendulum from polypharmacy to undertreatment. (See the figure below.)

We know how dangerous medical pendulum swings can be because we recently witnessed one: when health-care providers began to perceive that pain was under-treated, we swung the pendulum so hard that we mired ourselves in a deadly opioid crisis. We need to settle into the sweet spot—the fulcrum of medication balance—as we try to move away from a culture of polypharmacy. It is so important to remember that deprescribing does not mean eliminating all medications or that most medications are no longer needed. Deprescribing is not all or nothing. It's a process, a methodology that should be individualized. Deprescribing to optimize takes time, follow-through, and monitoring. Sometimes it might even require a restart to get it right.

Prescribing Pendulum

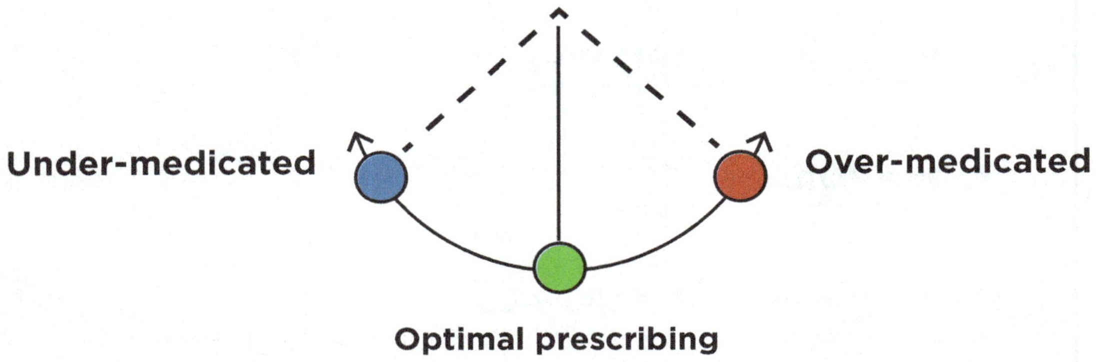

Proactive Approach

We grew up learning "a stitch in time saves nine," that successful businesses are proactive instead of reactive, and that fixing something earlier rather than later can save a lot of money and disruption. Let's take the same approach with our bodies! Medications can be needed to treat health conditions or to prevent further progression of a health condition. But medications can sometimes cause problems, too, and may eventually need to be stopped or reduced or changed. A proactive approach to deprescribing can prevent falls, accidents, and hospitalizations.

Individuals should get started now making a ***MedStrong Medication Optimization Plan (MOP)***, using the many resources provided throughout the workbook and in the

Resources section of this book. Providers should consider deprescribing before a patient suffers a fall or accident or debilitating side effect.

Every encounter between a patient and health-care provider is an opportunity to reduce unnecessary medications.[32]

That statement is probably my favorite takeaway from my research into deprescribing, and I hope that deprescribing soon becomes as much a part of our health-care culture as prescribing is now. Several steps are considered routine parts of meeting with a health-care provider today. During physicals you are asked about falling, wearing seat belts, and a host of other questions. Weight, height, and vitals are taken. Reviewing medications for need, safety, outcomes, and possible side effects should become routine practice too. Now is the time to take action!

Keeping Score

Date	Polypharmacy (# of medications)	AC Burden Score (page 36)	Frailty Score (page 55)

Overview of Part IV: The Way Forward

- Patients, caregivers, health-care providers, and pharmacists all play a role in polypharmacy, and all can play a role in fostering a culture of deprescribing to optimize medications.
- The Choosing Wisely Campaign can help patients avoid unnecessary medications.
- As deprescribing begins to be more accepted, we all have to work to make sure the pendulum does not swing too far toward undermedicating patients.
- The **MedStrong Optimization Plan (MOP)** and the variety of checklists and forms in this book can help patients and providers begin a deprescribing process.

It's time for patients, caregivers, health-care providers, pharmacists, and every part of the health-care infrastructure to take action against the hazards of polypharmacy and begin deprescribing to optimize for health and well-being.

Become part of the cultural shift to deprescribe.
Be empowered to start the conversation.

<u>D</u>eprescribe to <u>O</u>ptimize—**DO!**
Be ***MedStrong!***

Glossary & Resources

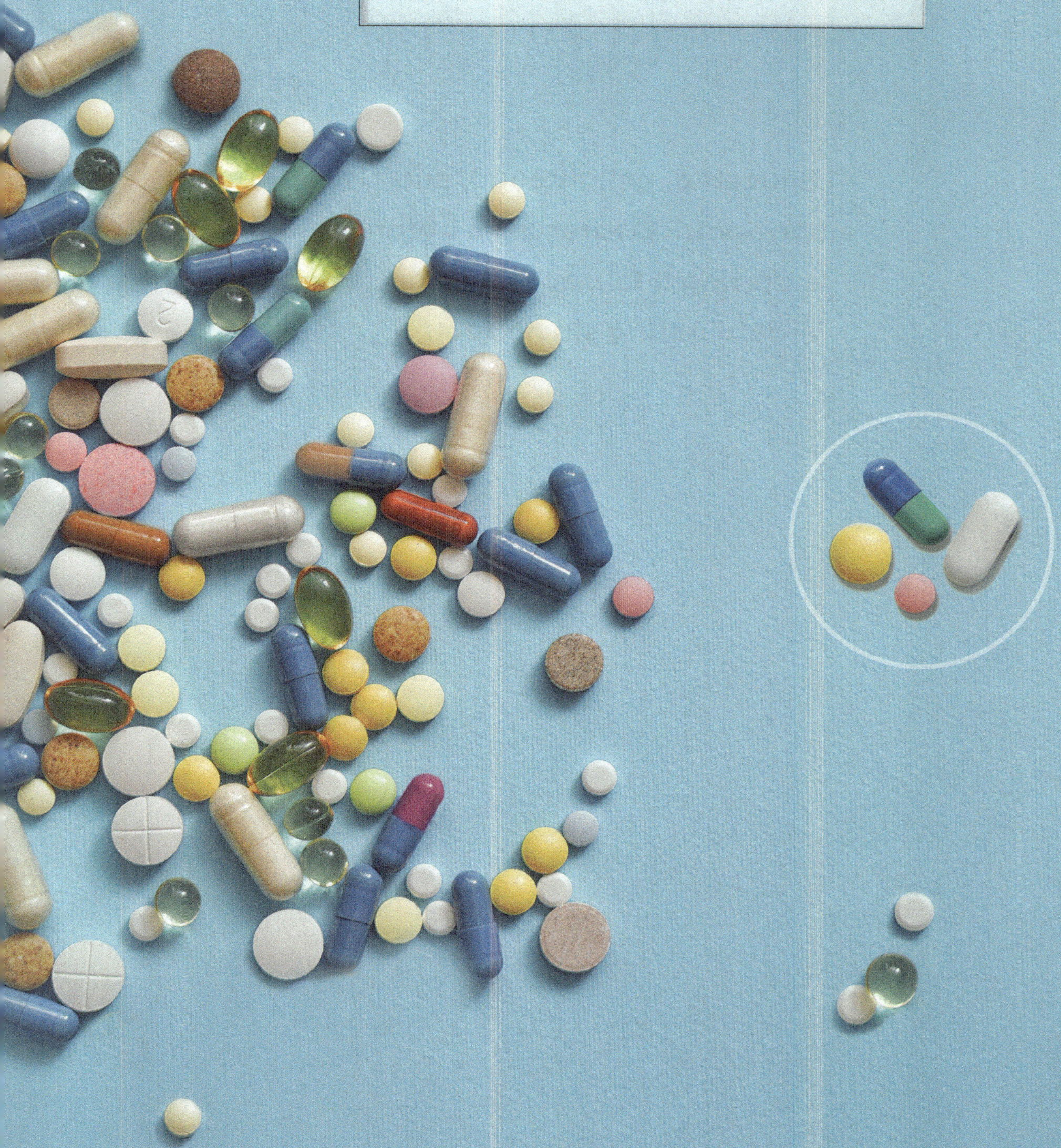

Educated, enlightened, and empowered! Deprescribe before suffering a fall, accident, or debilitating side effect.

Classes of Medications

Class/Family of Medication	Generic Names
Anticholinergics used for	
urinary incontinence	oxybutynin, solifenacin, tolterodine
COPD	aclidinium, ipratropium, tiotropium, umeclidinium
parkinsonism	benztropine
stomach spasm	dicyclomine, hyoscyamine
motion sickness, nausea, vomiting	scopolamine
Antidepressants	
SSRIs	fluoxetine, paroxetine, sertraline, citalopram, escitalopram
SNRIs	duloxetine, venlafaxine
TCAs	amitriptyline, nortriptyline
Others	bupropion, mirtazapine, trazodone
Antihistamines	
First Generation	brompheniramine, chlorpheniramine, clemastine, diphenhydramine, doxylamine, meclizine
Second Generation	cetirizine, fexofenadine, loratadine
Antipsychotics	
Second Generation	aripiprazole, clozapine, iloperidone, lurasidone, olanzapine, paliperidone, pimavanserin, quetiapine, risperidone, ziprasidone
First Generation	haloperidol
Antiseizure	
Hydantoin	phenytoin
Miscellaneous	carbamazepine, lamotrigine, levetiracetam, oxcarbazepine, topiramate, valproic acid, zonisamide
Benzodiazepines	
alprazolam, clonazepam, diazepam, lorazepam, oxazepam, temazepam, triazolam	
Bisphosphonates	
alendronate, ibandronate, risedronate, zolendronic acid	

Blood Pressure Medications	
ACE inhibitors	benazepril, captopril, enalapril, lisinopril, quinapril
ARBs	irbesartan, losartan, olmesartan, valsartan
Beta-blockers	atenolol, metoprolol, nebivolol
Calcium channel blockers	amlodipine, diltiazem, verapamil
Diuretics:	
Loop	bumetanide, ethacrynic acid, furosemide, torsemide
Potassium-sparing	amiloride, eplerenone, spironolactone, triamterene
Thiazide	chlorthalidone, hydrochlorothiazide

Dementia Medications	
Acetylcholinesterase inhibitors	donepezil, galantamine, rivastigmine
NMDA receptor antagonist	memantine

Diabetes Medications	
Biguanide	metformin
DDP-4 inhibitors	linagliptin, saxagliptin, sitagliptin
GLP-1	dulaglutide, exenatide, liraglutide, semaglutide
Insulin	insulin-aspart, -degludec, -detemir, -glargine, -lispro, -NPH, regular
Meglitinide	nateglinide, repaglinide
SGLT2 inhibitor	canagliflozin, dapagliflozin, empagliflozin
Sulfonylureas	glipizide, glyburide, glimepiride
Thiazolidinedione	pioglitazone, rosiglitazone

Eye Drops for Glaucoma	
Carbonic anhydrase inhibitors	brinzolamide, dorzolamide
Beta blocker	timolol
Prostaglandin analog	bimatoprost, latanoprost, travoprost

GABA analog
gabapentin, pregabalin

NSAIDs
diclofenac, ibuprofen, naproxen, meloxicam

Proton Pump Inhibitors (PPIs)
dexlansoprazole, esomeprazole, lansoprazole, omeprazole, pantoprazole, rabeprazole

Statins
atorvastatin, fluvastatin, lovastatin, pitavastatin, pravastatin, rosuvastatin, simvastatin

Glossary

Absorption: The ability of medicine to transfer from the gut to the bloodstream.

ACE inhibitors (angiotensin-converting enzyme inhibitors): A family of medicine used to treat high blood pressure. Adverse drug event: A harmful outcome to a medication. Agent: Another word for medication or drug.

Anticholinergics: Medications that are used to treat urinary incontinence. These medications can cause very drying effects. Other medications also have anticholinergic side effects, which can cause fast heart rate, cognition changes, and increased risk of falls.

Antiplatelet medications: A family of medicines that reduce the effects of platelets to reduce the risk of blood clots.

ARBs (Angiotensin II receptor blockers): A family of medicines used to treat high blood pressure. Examples include: losartan, valsartan, irbesartan, candesartan.

Benzodiazepines: A family of medicines used for anxiety. Examples are lorazepam, oxazepam, triazolam, alprazolam, clonazepam.

Bisphosphonates: A family of medications used to treat osteoporosis (brittle bones).

Chronic disease: A health condition that one lives with and potentially treats to reduce worsening of condition overtime or to reduce symptoms of the condition over time.

Citalopram: A medication used to treat depression and anxiety. Clinical inertia: Knowing there is a potential problem but not knowing how or when to take action such as deprescribing.

Cognitive bias: Thinking more subjectively, based on one's experience, than objectively, around the current circumstances or situation.

Comorbidity: More than one health condition that a person may have.

COPD (chronic obstructive pulmonary disease): Lung condition that causes difficulty with breathing, often due to smoking and other irritant exposure or chronic asthma.

COX-2-Inhibitor: A family of medications that is used for pain and inflammation. An example is celecoxib.

Culture of health care: The behaviors and expectations that society has regarding the practice of health care.

Deprescribing: The act or process of thoughtfully reducing, switch- ing, or stopping medications that may be inappropriate or no longer necessary.

Diphenhydramine: An over-the-counter antihistamine medication used to treat allergies and allergic reactions. It is also used in cough and cold medications and in medications to help one sleep.

Distribution: The pathway of a drug throughout the body systems.

Diuretic: A type of medication used to eliminate fluid, sometimes called a "water pill." Can be used for edema (such as swollen ankles), high blood pressure, and heart failure.

Drug-disease interaction: When a medication causes another health condition to worsen.

Drug-drug interaction: When one or more medications cause another medication to not work as expected.

Drug-food interaction: When a medication interferes with the expected outcome of a medication.

Elimination: The removal of a drug from the body through urine and feces.

Falls: The unintentional act of landing on the ground.

Formulary: List of medications covered by an insurance company or available at a facility such as a hospital.

Gabapentin: Medication that was originally used to treat seizures and is more commonly used for nerve-type pain, including neuropathy.

Glipizide: A medication used to treat diabetes.

Glyburide: A medication used to treat diabetes.

HbA1c: A blood test that determines the average blood sugar over 3 months.

Heart failure: A health condition where the heart is unable to pump blood as well or fill as well. There are many stages of this condition.

High-risk medications: Medications that have an increased chance of becoming toxic and causing harm instead of benefit.

Hydrochlorothiazide (HCTZ): A type of diuretic ("water pill").

Hypoglycemia: Low blood sugar.

Indication: The condition that a medication is being used for.

Isosorbide: A type of medication in the nitrate family used for angina; there are two forms: isosorbide dinitrate and isosorbide mononitrate.

Medication therapy management (MTM): A step-by-step process of reviewing a patient's medications, identifying possible medication-related problems, and determining an action plan to reduce problems.

Metabolism: The chemical changes of a medication within the body necessary to activate the medication and/or make it so that the medication can be eliminated.

NSAIDs (nonsteroidal anti-inflammatory drugs): A family of medicines used to treat pain and inflammation. Examples are ibuprofen, naproxen, diclofenac, indomethacin.

Optimize: To maximize benefit and reduce harm with the least amount of medications, with the lowest appropriate dose, at the correct frequency, while monitoring for appropriate and best outcomes.

Orthostatic hypotension: A drop in blood pressure when changing position—for example, sitting to standing.

Overmedication: The excessive or inappropriate use or continuation of unnecessary medication.

Pharmacodynamics: What the drug does to a body, its actions and side effects.

Pharmacokinetics: What the body does to a drug: absorption, distribution, metabolism, and elimination.

Polypharmacy: Multiple medications, typically five or more, that a person takes.

Potentially inappropriate medications: Medications that pose more harm than benefit or may be unnecessary.

Potentially inappropriate prescribing: Prescribing of high-risk medications, unnecessary medications, or medications to treat a side effect rather than addressing the problem-causing drug, when another, safer option may be used.

Prescribing-cascade: The use of medication to treat the side effects of another medication.

Proton pump inhibitors (PPI): Medications used to treat stomach acid problems such as GERD, or gastric esophageal reflux disorder.

Readmission: Having to be hospitalized again soon after being discharged from a hospital, typically within 30 days.

Shared decision-making: When patient and prescribers discuss patient goals and therapy goals and reach a decision on treatment (or nontreatment) of a condition together.

Simvastatin: A medication used to treat cholesterol.

Statins: A family of medicines used to treat high cholesterol. Examples are atorvastatin, simvastatin, rosuvastatin.

Telehealth: A way in which health-care professionals can communicate long-distance with a patient, typically via the phone or computer audio and video.

Tramadol: A medication in the opioid family that is used for pain.

Transitions of care: A shift in responsibility of care for an individual from place to place; for example from hospital to home.

Treatment guidelines: An algorithm to treat a health condition grounded in evidence-based medicine and decided upon through a panel of experts.

Z-drugs: A family of medicines used as sleep aids. Examples include zolpidem, zopiclone, eszopiclone, zaleplon.

Zolpidem: A medication used to treat insomnia.

Resources

American Geriatrics Society (AGS) (https://www.americangeriatrics.org) (https://www.americangeriatrics.org/publications-tools/ patient-education)

The home of The Beers Criteria, which highlight medications that could be potentially inappropriate in patients.

American Geriatrics Society's Health in Aging Foundation (www.Healthinaging.org)

The Health in Aging website offers a number of information sheets for the health-care consumer to view, including "Ten Medications Older Adults Should Avoid or Use with Caution."

American Society of Consultant Pharmacists (ASCP) Foundation (https://www.ascp.com/page/foundation) and American Society of Consultant Pharmacists (ASCP) Foundation (https://www.ascp.com)

Provides a website called Help With My Meds (helpwithmymeds.org) (https://www.ascp.com/mpage/Care_Pharmacist) that can help users find a senior-care pharmacist in your area. Board- certified geriatric pharmacists are available in every state, Canada, and Australia.

Anticholinergic Burden Calculator (http://www.acbcalc.com) This calculator helps to calculate and find a score for medications that can cause anticholinergic effects, including dry effects, confusion, fast heartbeat, and falls.

Chronic Heart Failure Action Plan (https://assets.heartfoundation. org.nz/documents/shop/heart-healthcare/non-stock-resources/heart- failure-action-plan.pdf)

My Heart Failure Action Plan by Heart Foundation provides a daily check-in and action guide to monitor heart failure to help maintain a better quality of life and prevent hospitalization.

Chronic Obstructive Pulmonary Disease (COPD) Action Plan

(https://www.lung.org/getmedia/c7657648-a30f-4465-af92- fc762411922e/fy20-ala-copd-action-plan.pdf)

My COPD Action Plan by the American Lung Association provides a daily check-in and action guide to monitor COPD to help maintain a better quality of life and prevent hospitalization.

Choosing Wisely (https://www.choosingwisely.org/societies/ american-geriatrics-society/)

Choosing Wisely, a program offered through the American Board of Internal Medicine, highlights several concerns that we should heed as health-care consumers. Though it is intended to be a guide for prescribers, individuals can review it to help start conversations with providers.

Clinical Frailty Scale (https://www.dal.ca/sites/gmr/our-tools/clini- cal-frailty-scale.html)

This scale shows varying levels of frailty from very fit to end of life. Challenge yourself to move up the scale for better quality of life and health.

The Comprehensive Geriatric Assessment

(https://www.cgakit.com/cga)

Assessment toolkits for health-care professionals to assess and evalu- ate older adults on quality of life, mobility, and fall prevention.

Deprescribing.org

This Canadian program is actively reviewing deprescribing. The organization has begun to review and provide algorithms to deprescribe or reduce medications such as benzodiazepines, proton pump inhibitors, antiseizure medications, and antidiabetic medications.

Drive to Deprescribe (https://paltc.org/drive2deprescribe) Programming available for facilities and health-care professionals to institute education and goals of reducing and optimizing medications in post-acute and long-term care settings.

Drugs.com

Website available for learning about medications (both prescription and nonprescription), checking potential drug interactions, and identifying pills.

Lown Institute (https://lowninstitute.org/reports/medication-over- load-americas-other-drug-problem/)

Lown Institute is a think tank that advocates for a "just and caring system for health." The publications are thorough and provide great ideas, examples, and statistics.

Medstopper (http://medstopper.com)

This website can help identify potentially inappropriate medications and the priority in which one may want to consider deprescribing medication.

Mini Mental Status Examination (MMSE)

(https://www.dementiacarecentral.com/mini-mental-state-exam/) This website provides the MMSE along with a host of information for people caring for those with dementia.

STOPPFall (Screening Tool of Older Persons Prescriptions in older adults with high fall risk) (https://academic.oup.com/ageing/ article/50/4/1189/6043386)

This tool considers whether withdrawal of a medication should be considered for potential adverse events, especially if a person is at a high risk of falls.

Stopping Elderly Accidents, Deaths, and Injuries (STEADI)

(https://www.cdc.gov/steadi/index.html)

This program from the Centers for Disease Control (CDC) aims to help prevent falls. It educates individuals and health-care professionals about screening for and preventing falls, accidents, and injuries that can lead to death in older adults. There are many options to choose from for information on preventing falls, including SAFE:

- Screen for medications that could increase falls, injuries, or accidents;
- Assess for the best treatment for the individual's active health conditions;
- Formulate an action plan to optimize treatment; and
- Educate the individual and caregiver on medication changes and reducing falls, accidents, and injuries.

WISE & WELL Dr. Donna Bartlett (https://donnabartlett.com) This website is dedicated to learning more about deprescribing.

Endnotes

1. Rankin A, Cadogan CA, Patterson SM, et al. Interventions to improve the appropriate use of polypharmacy for older people. *Cochrane Database Syst Rev.* 2018;(9):CD008165.
2. Reeve E, Gnjidic D, Long J, Hilmer S. A systematic review of the emerging definition of 'deprescribing' with network analysis: implications for future research and clinical practice. *Br J Clin Pharmacol.* 2015;80(6):1254–1268. doi:10.1111/bcp.1273
3. Scott IA, Gray LC, Martin JH, et al. Deciding when to stop: towards evidence-based deprescribing of drugs in older adults. *Evid Based Med.* 2013;18(4):121–124.
4. Hajjar ER, Gray SL, Slattum PW, et al. Geriatrics. In *Pharmacotherapy: A Pathophysiological Approach.* 9th ed. McGraw-Hill Education, 2014.
5. Hajjar ER, Hanlon JT. Polypharmacy in elderly patients. *Am J Geriatr Pharmacother.* 2007;5(4):345–351.
6. National Institute on Alcohol Abuse and Alcoholism. Harmful interactions: mixing alcohol with medicines. Updated November 2020. Accessed March 10, 2022. https://www.niaaa.nih.gov/sites/default/files/publications/NIAAA_Harmful_Interactions_English.pdf
7. McGrath K, Hajjar ER, Kumar C, Hwang C, Salzman B. Deprescribing: a simple method for reducing polypharmacy. *J Fam Pract.* 2017;66(7):436–445.
8. Brookes L. Easy to start, hard to stop: polypharmacy and deprescribing. *Medscape.* Jun 1, 2017.
9. Scott IA, Hilmer SN, Reeve E, et al. Reducing inappropriate polypharmacy: the process of deprescribing. *JAMA Inter Med.* 2015;175(5):827–834.
10. Farrell B, Mangin D. Deprescribing is an essential part of good prescribing. *Am Fam Physician.* 2019;99(1):7–9.
11. Scott IA, Hilmer SN, Reeve E, et al. Reducing inappropriate polypharmacy: the process of deprescribing. *JAMA Inter Med.* 2015;175(5):827–834.
12. Iyer S, Naganathan V, McLachlan AL, Le Couteur DG. Medication withdrawal trials in people age 65 years and older: a systematic review. *Drugs Aging.* 2008;25(12)1021–1031.
13. Van der Cammen TJM, Rajkumar C, Onder G, et al. Drug cessation in complex older adults: time for action. *Age Ageing.* 2014;43(1):20–25.

14 Tannenbaum C, Martin P, Tamblyn R, et al. Reduction of inappropriate benzodiazepine prescriptions among older adults through direct patient education: the EMPOWER cluster randomized trial. *JAMA Intern Med.* 2014;174(6):890–898.15

15. American Heart Association Scientific Sessions 2020, Presentation MP269 Black patients less likely to receive added, higher dose meds to control blood pressure. Newsroom. November 9, 2020. https://newsroom.heart.org/news/black-patients-less-likely-to-receive-added-higher-dose-meds-to-control-blood-pressure
16. Farrell B, Mangin D. Deprescribing is an essential part of good prescribing. *American Family Physician.* 2019;99(1):7–9.

17. Rea F, Biffi A, Ronco R, et al. Cardiovascular outcomes and mortality associated with discontinuing statins in older patients receiving polypharmacy. *JAMA Network Open*. 2021;4(6):e2113186.
18. Giral P, et al. Cardiovascular effect of discontinuing statins for primary prevention at the age of 75 years: a nationwide population-based cohort study in France. Eur Heart J. 2019;40(43): 3516–3525.
19. Reeve E, Thompson W, Farrell B. Deprescribing: a narrative review of the evidence and practical recommendations for recognizing opportunities and taking action. E*ur J Intern Med.* 2017;38:3–11.
20. Parker B, Thompson P. Effect of statins on skeletal muscle: exercise, myopathy, and muscle outcomes. *Exerc Sport Sci Rev.* 2012;40(4):188–194.
21. By the 2019 American Geriatrics Society Beers Criteria® Update Expert Panel. American Geriatrics Society 2019 Updated AGS Beers Criteria® for Potentially Inappropriate Medication Use in Older Adults. *J Am Geriatr Soc.* 2019;67(4):674–694.
22. O'Mahony DO, O'Sullivan D, Byrne S, et al. STOPP/START criteria for potentially inappropriate prescribing in older people: version 2. *Age Ageing*. 2015;44(2):213–218. doi:10.1093/ageing/ afu145
23. STEADI Stopping Elderly Accidents, Deaths & Injuries – Older Adult Fall Prevention. Centers for Disease Control and Prevention, National Center for Injury Prevention and Control. Updated 2023. https://www.cdc.gov/steadi/index.html
24. Walker T. Pharmacist-Driven Intervention Program Reduces Readmissions Drug Topics Journal. 2019;163(1). https://www.drugtopics.com/view/pharmacist-driven-intervention-program-reduces-readmissions
25. Hanlon JT, Schmader KE, Samsa GP, et al. A method for assessing drug therapy appropriateness. J Clin Epidemiol. 1992;45(10):1045–51. doi:10.1016/0895-4356(92)90144-c . PMID: 1474400.
26. Hanlon JT, Schmader KE. The medication appropriateness index at 20: where it started, where it has been, and where it may be going. *Drugs Aging.* 2013;30(11):893–900. doi:10.1007/s40266-013–0118–4 . PMID: 24062215; PMCID: PMC3831621.
27. Brookes L. Deprescribing benzodiazepines: changing attitudes. *Medscape.* June 15, 2018. https://www.medscape.com/viewarticle/897919_1
28. Duraisingham S, Jubraj B, Marvin V, et al. Stopping inappropriate medicines in the outpatient setting. *GM.* 2015;(April):35–41.
29. Brookes L. Deprescribing benzodiazepines: changing attitudes. *Medscape.* June 15, 2018. https://www.medscape.com/viewarticle/897919_1
30. Scott IA, Hilmer SN, Reeve E, et al. Reducing inappropriate polypharmacy: the process of deprescribing. *JAMA Inter Med.* 2015;175(5):827–834.
31. Bean RB. *Sir William Osler: Aphorisms from His Bedside Teachings & Writings.* New York: Henry Schuman, 1950.
32. Mishori R. What needs to change to make deprescribing doable. *Fam Pract Manag.* 2018;25(3):5–6.
33. Brookes L. Deprescribing benzodiazepines: changing attitudes. *Medscape.* June 15, 2018. https://www.medscape.com/ viewarticle/897919_1

MedStrong Forms

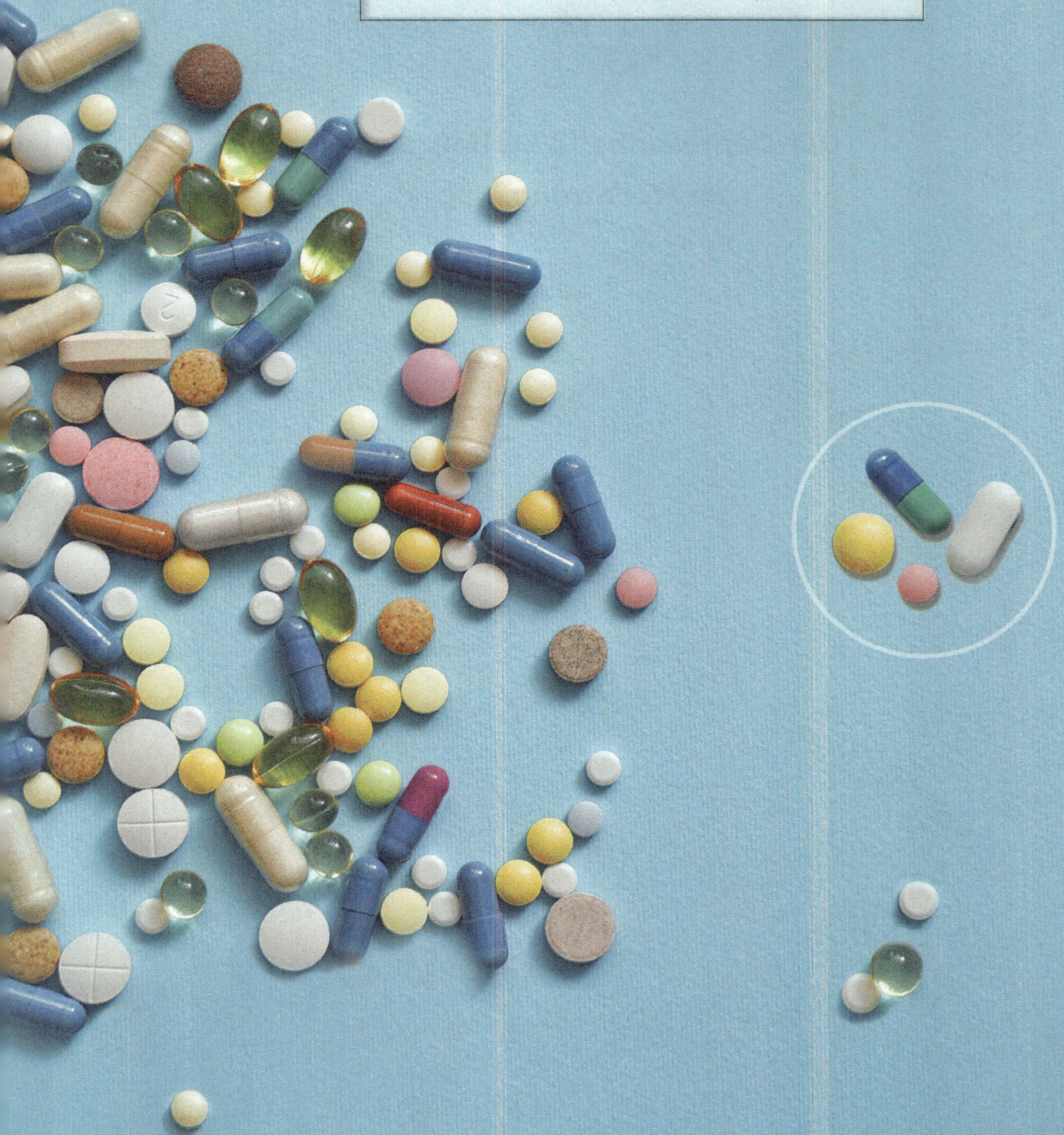

DO–Deprescribe to Optimize!

Be *MedStrong*!

MedStrong Prescription Medication List

PRESCRIPTION Name of Prescription Medication and Strength of Dose	How Taken	Reason for Taking	Does the Problem Still Exist?	Is the Medical Condition Controlled?
1.				
2.				
3.				
4.				
5.				
6.				
7.				
8.				
9.				
10.				
11.				
12.				
13.				
14.				
15.				
16.				
17.				
18.				
19.				
20.				
21.				

MedStrong OVER-THE-COUNTER Medication List

OVER THE COUNTER OTC Medication, Supplement, or Herbal and Strength of Dose	How Taken	Reason for Taking	Does the Problem Still Exist?	Is the Medical Condition Controlled?
1.				
2.				
3.				
4.				
5.				
6.				
7.				
8.				
9.				
10.				
11.				
12.				
13.				
14.				
15.				
16.				
17.				
18.				
19.				
20.				
21.				

Prescription Medications

- Look at the Medication List you just made. Are there question marks? Uncertainties?
- Formulate questions around these unknowns. List your questions here:

PRESCRIPTION MEDICATION	Question

Over the Counter Medications

- Are you taking OTCs, supplements, vitamins, herbals?
- What are you trying to treat?
- What are you hoping to alleviate or how are you thinking you benefit from the product?`

NON-PRESCRIPTIONS	Purpose	Question

MedStrong QUESTION LIST

Check the questions, to ask your health-care providers, that fit your concerns.

Questions to Ask Yourself

- ☐ Am I having problems paying for all of my prescriptions?
- ☐ Do I sometimes choose which medicines to take or not take because of affordability issues?
- ☐ Do I take some or all of my medications differently than how they were prescribed to "stretch them out"? For example, do I take a pill every other day even if it is prescribed to take daily?

Questions to Ask Your Health-Care Provider

- ☐ Are there any medications that I am currently taking that may no longer be necessary?
- ☐ Are there any medications that may be dosed too high for my age, health status, kidney function, or with other medications I am taking?
- ☐ Could one of my health concerns actually be a side effect of a medication?
- ☐ Are there safer medications I could be taking?
- ☐ Can any of my medications increase my risk of falls?
- ☐ Can any combination of these medications increase my risk of falls or increase a risk of bleeding?

Questions to Ask at the Pharmacy

- ☐ Could I be using an OTC product to treat a side effect of one of my prescription medications?
- ☐ Is this OTC product okay to take with my current medications and my health conditions?
- ☐ Are any of my medications potentially being prescribed for a side effect of another prescription (prescribing cascade)?
- ☐ Could any of my medications increase my risk of falling? If so, which ones?
- ☐ If I could take fewer medications, which ones should I ask my doctor about possibly stopping?
- ☐ Am I taking any unnecessary medications?
- ☐ How long will it take for this medication to start working as it should?
- ☐ Is this a medication that I need to fill regularly?
- ☐ When would be the best time of day to take this medication?
- ☐ Is it possible for you to help me figure out a schedule to take my medications?

Questions to Ask When an Older Adult Is Hospitalized

- [ ] Could any of my medications—prescription, OTC, herbal, or supplements—have contributed to this condition?
- [ ] Could my medications have interacted to have caused my hospitalization, such as medications that have additive effects / side effects?
- [ ] Are there any of my current medications that might be unnecessary or that you think we should discuss with the primary care physician or specialist?
- [ ] Are there any medications, OTCs, or supplements that may be interacting with blood tests or any other tests or procedures?

____

____

____

Questions to Ask When Being Discharged from the Hospital

- [ ] Are there changes to my medications or how I should take them?
- [ ] Are there medications that are similar to medications that I take at home? I do not want to duplicate my medications.
- [ ] Are there any medications I should no longer take?
- [ ] How long should I continue taking any new medications?

Are some just for a short period of time or just when needed?

____

____

____

My Questions about Specific Concerns or Specific Medications

____

Each area of health care is a possible setting to ask about your medications:

- **At the Pharmacy**
- **At the MD's Office**
- **At the Specialist**
- **At the Hospital**
- **At the NP and PA Office**
- **At the Short-term Rehab**
- **At the Long-term Care Facility**
- **At the Dentist**
- **At the Optometrist**
- **At the Physical Therapist**
- **At the Occupational Therapist**
- **With Hospice and Palliative Care Teams**

Shared Decision-Making with Your Physician

If you are uncertain what to do regarding your medications or you have a choice:

- ASK: What would you do if you were me? (This is an acceptable question, but it does not need to be the ultimate decision.)
- List the pros and cons to help you decide.

Medication ______________________________

PROS	CONS

Medication ______________________________

PROS	CONS

Medication ______________________________

PROS	CONS

MedStrong Deprescribing Form

Medication: ______________________________ Date: ____________________

Why is this medication being deprescribed? ________________________________

DEPRESCRIBE INSTRUCTIONS:

Changed to: __________ Reduced to: __________ Stopped: Date: ______________

Taper: ☐ Yes ☐ No If yes, taper instructions: ____________________________

____

MONITOR:

Labs: _____________________ Date: ________________________________

Check: ____________________ and keep a log. ___________________________

(Examples: blood pressure, heart rate, blood glucose, weight)

Date: _________ Time: _________ Results: _______________________________

HOW DO I FEEL?:

☐ No different: ____

☐ Not so good because: ____

☐ Better, I notice that: ____

FOLLOW-UP WITH:

Name of health care provider: ____

Phone number: ____

Date of next appointment: ____

MedStrong Medication Change Form

Medication and Strength	How Many, How Often	Prescribed by	Date/ Year Started	Still Taking?	Date Medication Stopped or Changed	Medication Restarted or Changed, Why?

About the Author

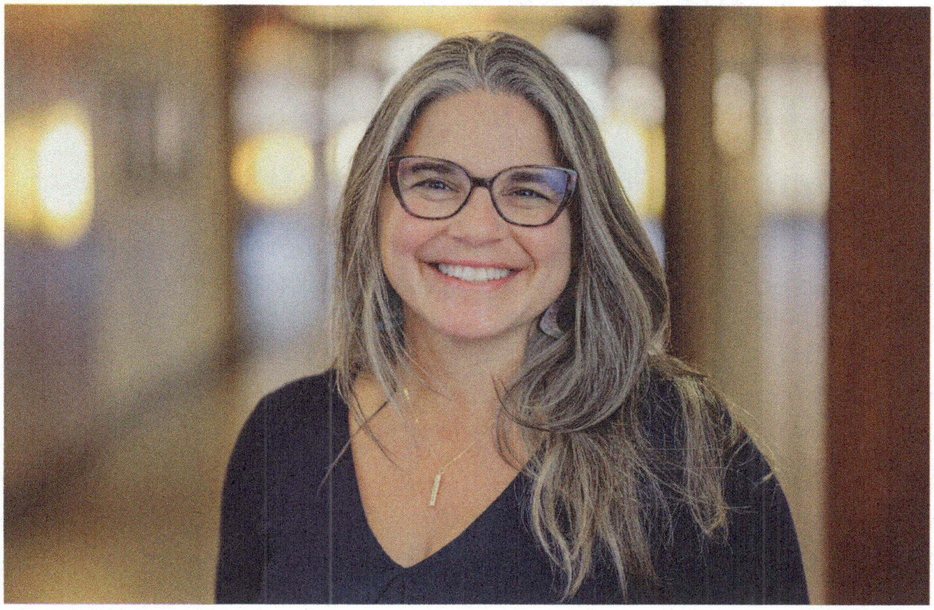

DR. DONNA BARTLETT is a Board-Certified Geriatric Pharmacist licensed in Massachusetts. Currently, Dr. Bartlett is a Professor of Pharmacy Practice at the Massachusetts College of Pharmacy and Health Sciences University, and oversees an internal medicine clinical site at a local hospital. Dr. Bartlett has over 17 years' experience as a clinical pharmacist and over 20 years of retail experience. She served on many boards including Pharmacy and Therapeutics Committee, the MA Falls Prevention Coalition, and the Advisory Committee of the Regional Center for Poison Control and Prevention Serving Massachusetts and Rhode Island. Dr. Bartlett has presented locally, regionally, nationally, and internationally, and presented at the first International Deprescribing Conference in Denmark in the fall of 2022.

Education expertise and areas of interest includes polypharmacy, deprescribing, geriatrics, medication access and affordability, and falls prevention. Dr. Bartlett cohosts the podcast *The Med List* and hosts her own website dedicated to deprescribing WISE & WELL Dr. Donna Bartlett **https://donnabartlett.com** She is the author of *MedStrong: Shed Your Meds for a Better, Healthier You-Aging Well through Deprescribing*. Donna and her husband have two children and live in Paxton, MA.

MedStrong

Shed Your Meds for a Better, Healthier You

Companion to the *MedStrong* Workbook

by Donna Bartlett, PharmD, BCGP

Medications can keep us healthy and strong, and are often truly life-saving. Yet, as we age, the body naturally changes, along with its ability to absorb, metabolize and eliminate medication. Here's the truth about "aging conditions" such as forgetfulness, confusion, insomnia, weakness, and falling—many of these conditions can be linked directly to overprescribing of medications.

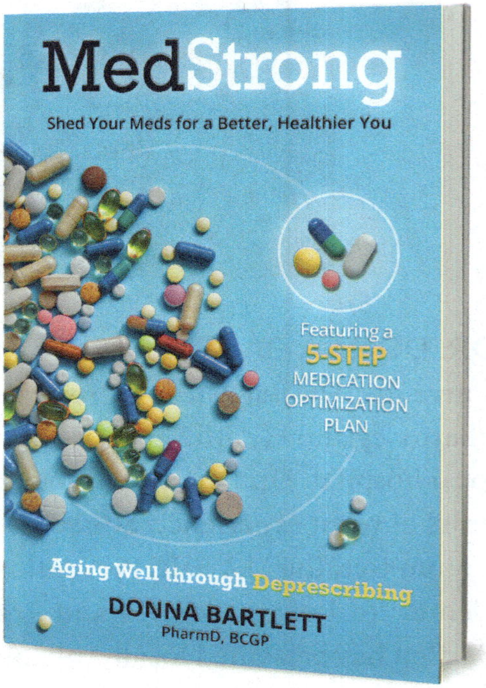

Dr. Donna Bartlett is a practicing, board-certified geriatric pharmacist with decades of witnessing the enormous suffering and compromised quality of life wreaked by overmedication. She is a leading authority on "deprescribing"—the evidence-based process of reducing, switching, or stopping medications.

Packed with countless real-world examples and extensive medical data and research—translated into "everyday" language—***MedStrong*** is your guide to safely optimize your list of prescription and over-the-counter medications.

Ready to boost the quality of your life by taking only the meds you need, and in the right doses for you? Let ***MedStrong*** be your guide to becoming an educated healthcare consumer—one empowered to create a better, healthier you!

Published by WELLhood Publishing

ISBN-978-1737756309 | 252 pages | $ 19.00

Kindle | $9.99

Available at Amazon.com and other booksellers

Notes

Made in the USA
Coppell, TX
11 October 2026

92519830R00066